HEALTHCARE
FOR LESS

HEALTHCARE FOR LESS

Getting the Care You Need—
Without Breaking the Bank

MICHELLE KATZ, M.S.N.

Foreword by R. Martin Bashir, M.D.

healthyliving**books**

New York • London

A HEALTHY LIVING BOOK
Published by
Hatherleigh Press
5-22 46th Avenue, Suite 200
Long Island City, NY 11101
www.hatherleighpress.com

Library of Congress Cataloging-in-Publication Data

Katz, Michelle.
  Healthcare for less : getting the care you need without breaking the bank
/ Michelle Katz.
    p. cm.
  "A Healthy Living book."
  ISBN-13: 978-1-57826-222-9
  ISBN-10: 1-57826-222-4
  1. Medical care. 2. Insurance, Health. 3. Physician and patient. I.
Title.
  RA410.K38 2006
  362.1--dc22

                        2006002114

Healthy Living Books are available for bulk purchase, special promotions, and premiums. For information on reselling and special purchase opportunities, please call us at 800-528-2550 and ask for the Special Sales Manager.

Disclaimer

This book is for informational and educational purposes only, and it is not a substitute for the professional medical or legal advice given to you by your attorney, your physician, or any other professional advisers.

Using this book should not substitute for the advice of a physician and does not create a doctor-patient relationship. You are strongly advised to follow the advice of your physician, pharmacists, and other healthcare providers who know the specifics of your medical condition. Do not use any information in this book without first consulting your healthcare providers.

The patients and characters in this book are based on real patients or events, but their names and details have been changed.

Cover design by Deborah Miller
Interior design by Deborah Miller and Jacinta Monniere

10 9 8 7 6 5 4 3 2 1
Printed in Canada

Dedicated to all those who pay too much for healthcare.

Acknowledgments

AS A HEALTHCARE CONSULTANT in the media with a Masters degree in nursing, I have had a great opportunity to put my finger on the pulse of healthcare in America.

Through my clinical and administrative experiences in the healthcare industry, as well as my own struggle with medical care costs, I have gained a greater understanding on how to become a smart healthcare consumer and began sharing that information with others; from students, to CEOs, to physicians and politicians (including my grandmother and her friends on programs that seem too complicated for the elderly such as Medicare and Medicaid). My insight has helped others endure my plight on a daily basis, and resulted in this book: *Healthcare for Less.*

I am thankful to all who supported me throughout this arduous process, especially those who shared their medical billing knowledge, successes and failures, with me, including Montgomery General Hospital, William Mac-Cartee, and Thomas Scully. Also, I would like to thank those politicians who were eager to lend an ear and share their stories, but are constrained by our own democracy. I am very grateful to my publisher, Kevin Moran, who encouraged me to write this book and his entire patient, yet enthusiastic staff at Hatherleigh Press, who dealt with the constant changes in healthcare as the book was being written.

Finally, and most importantly, my deepest thanks go to my husband, Roshan Martin. Without his inspiration, love, knowledge, and support, I could not have written this book.

Foreword

W E ARE ON THE VERGE OF THE greatest healthcare crisis in American history. Over 50 million Americans are living without health insurance, taking their lives into their own hands. Healthcare costs are spiraling out of control with no relief in sight, despite insurance companies annually lowering reimbursement to doctors and hospitals, while keeping a larger piece of the pie for themselves. The "baby boomer" generation is aging and developing healthcare needs, creating a demand on the supply of services available. This, along with the fact that we already have a crippling nursing shortage in the U.S., is driving up costs to maintain hospitals, many of which are on the verge of bankruptcy. Medical malpractice premiums are at an all-time high, largely due to the lack of a "cap" on malpractice claims, forcing physicians to practice "defensive" medicine by ordering excessive, expensive tests. Some doctors are leaving practice due to the outrageous malpractice insurance costs, creating a void in specialties such as OB-GYN and family medicine. As a result, major healthcare insurers have driven up premiums to pay for these elevated outpatient and inpatient healthcare costs.

What is an American to do to ensure that they receive good care, but not break the bank? Enter *Healthcare for Less*. Michelle Katz reaches the core of healthcare and educates the reader on fundamentally important topics in healthcare, enabling the patient to negotiate discounts with providers and insurers. How can a patient lower the balance due to their doctor or hospital? Is there room for negotiating? How does a patient approach their healthcare provider to write off unpaid bills? These questions are all answered in *Healthcare for Less,* a unique, ground-breaking reference that clearly explains difficult-to-understand aspects of healthcare. Katz outlines how the consumer can maximize the benefits of their insurance, understand the medical lingo, and then uncover errors in medical bills. She also explains the most important aspects of choosing a doctor and selecting healthcare insurance, focusing on ways to save money, including through preventative medicine. *Healthcare for Less* helps us all understand the complex, new Medicare Part D prescription plan, HSAs, and COBRA.

We are always seeking creative, cost-cutting, ways to save money in healthcare, but little is available about how to save and what to do. *Healthcare for Less* explains creative approaches to take when dealing with a physician, a hospital, an insurer, in order to receive discounts and even "courtesy" on unpaid bills. Is healthcare insurance a necessity? Is there really a difference between doctors and insurance plans? Do we all need to get insurance? How can we afford not to have it if we get sick? These are important questions we should all be asking and which *Healthcare for Less* answers eloquently.

One thing is clear: the cost of healthcare in America has become practically impossible to manage without insurance. The system is broken and needs to be fixed, but until then, *Healthcare for Less* can help us all understand how we can get good care without mortgaging the house in the process.

—*R. Martin Bashir, M.D., FACP, FACG*

Dr. R. Martin Bashir, author of over 40 original medical publications and national speaker on the latest medical technologies, is recognized as one of the nations Top Doctors*, a Fellow of the American College of Physicians and Fellow of the American College of Gastroenterology. He is a Clinical Assistant Professor and Attending Physician of Georgetown University Medical Center, Sibley Hospital, Washington Hospital Center, and Children's National Medical Center in Washington, D.C.

Washingtonian Magazine 2002–2006, US News and World Report, "Who's Who"

Contents

Introduction

W E ALL WILL, INEVITABLY, be confronted with the same dilemma: as we age, our bodies deteriorate and we get ill. Along the way, we likely will need the help of a doctor, nurse, and potentially even a hospital, to treat our diseases. Our population is aging and living longer, largely as a result of the advances we have achieved in healthcare. However, as more Americans demand the latest technology and state-of-the-art treatments, healthcare will continue to be expensive. We will not accept the mediocre care offered by socialized systems, but we also do not want to pay too much for it. In our system, the available treatments and medicines will continue to improve and cost more. Moreover, the more healthcare that is available, the more expensive it becomes, and the more insurance has to cover.

We remain a nation in healthcare denial, expecting to live longer and not wanting to consider the healthcare expenses related to treating unexpected illness. Do we really need health insurance, we ask ourselves? Should we invest in our healthcare, or should we put ourselves at risk by not paying for health insurance because it is too expensive? Is there a way those of us who cannot afford the best healthcare can still receive excellent healthcare without mortgaging our houses or going bankrupt?

Unfortunately, the expense of good healthcare adds to the insurance confusion, since not everything is covered, even by some good policies. Insurance companies have figured out clever ways to avoid paying for care, despite raising our premiums. In our current healthcare system, it can be hard to determine just what our healthcare insurance covers. You might pay a flat rate for insurance and later be surprised when a bill is received for a service you thought you wouldn't have to pay for. Because there is no pressure placed upon the prices required by healthcare, there's no real incentive to provide you a better price. Because of that, costs go up, and insurance companies hand them down to you, making it even more difficult for some of us to have affordable healthcare.

In 2003, 15 percent of Americans were uninsured, up from 14.6 percent in 2002. While more than 80 percent of the uninsured are over age 65, the newest trend, and a more frightening one, is the amount of young and midlife adults without insurance. This number continues to rise and is an indication of where our healthcare system is headed.

Congress has tried to tackle our healthcare issues by suggesting refundable tax credits, capping medical malpractice awards, extending existing programs, privatizing public insurance, and attempting to establish a universal healthcare system. Unfortunately, all its attempts thus far have failed or have been lost in the legislative process.

There are some pending developmentst, however. In January 2004, President George W. Bush addressed the country on the rising cost of healthcare and discussed the creation of Health Savings Accounts. Some people believe HSAs will have a positive impact on the number of uninsured adults and may also reduce spending on unnecessary care. Medicare is the driving force behind healthcare insurance companies. More than often, if Medicare reimburses a certain way on a procedure, the insurance companies will follow. By signing this Medicare bill, the President moved us in the right direction, but the healthcare industry still has a long way to go.

So where is our healthcare system now? Some may say, "in a state of transition"; others may say, "a complete mess." Where does the healthcare system need to go? Tom Scully, the director of the Centers for Medicare & Medicaid Services (CMS), has said that there needs to be regulation on insurance companies, as well as a scale for the under-65 market. Getting to this point may take a long time. In early 2006, more insurance companies began offering Medicare benefits, but not all companies are following this pattern. The healthcare system is becoming even more confusing because of this. There are more options offered... or are there?

The most important thing is never to give the healthcare system control of your health. Take back control, and empower yourself with the tools to lower your healthcare costs. These tools are more readily available than you might think. For example, something as basic as strengthening your relationship with your doctor could save you annoyance, time, and money. By educating yourself on healthcare, you can establish a stronger patient/physician relationship and lower the cost of your health insurance.

PART I

BUILDING A RELATIONSHIP WITH YOUR DOCTOR

CHAPTER 1

How to Choose
a Doctor

C HOOSING THE RIGHT PHYSICIAN is one of the most important decisions you will make in your life and could mean the difference between life and death. You could argue that all physicians are the same, but that is far from the truth.

You can never spend too much time investigating a physician's background and credentials. Do so in advance, because it is always easier to cancel a first appointment than end a relationship with a doctor whom you have been seeing for basic checkups but who seems to be unable to handle more of your complex healthcare issues or, worse, does not seem interested in your healthcare questions. When choosing a physician, *remember:* it is your responsibility as the patient to make sure the doctor is an active participant in your healthcare plan. If this is assumed or overlooked, you may end up with a large, unnecessary bill.

I was once referred by a friend to a great obstetrician–gynecologist for a routine annual checkup and Pap smear; however, the $420 bill I received was far from routine, since I had failed to check whether she participated in my Cigna PPO health plan—a costly mistake on my part. It is often tempting to simply take the recommendation of a friend who refers a good physician. However, as I discovered the hard way, this can be expensive if the doctor is not a preferred provider in your health plan. That is where a good primary care physician can be invaluable. Usually, if your primary physician, or "gatekeeper," is a busy, well-qualified physician, the participating doctors he works with (to whom he refers his patients) will also be competent and, most importantly, will participate in your health plan. Remember to specify that you would like to be referred to specialists who participate in your health plan.

As you can see from the above, this was a costly mistake. I assumed that the doctor would accept my insurance but failed to realize that many doctors do not have the time to research every patient's insurance plan, and sometimes even the office staff does not have the time because they are busy caring for patients. Would you let an auto mechanic choose your car? That might not be a bad idea, but only you know what type of car you like; he or she might not have the same preferences as you and might prefer to work on a certain car. Which brings me to the next point: before you get into a situation where you need a doctor, do your research and choose the right doctor for you, one who participates in your health insurance plan. This may take a long time, but remember, this is your health we are talking about and you cannot turn in your health after a few years as you can a car. You are stuck with it for life, so you might as well be happy with the person who is going to help maintain it!

Choosing the Right "Gatekeeper"

Choosing a good primary care doctor is perhaps the most important step you can take to ensure that you get good medical care at a good price. A primary care doctor should be seen as your healthcare partner in the long haul, helping you to establish your health goals and periodically evaluating how you're doing while treating any illnesses that may come up along the way. Ideally, a primary care doctor can offer you the following benefits:

- **A good starting point in the healthcare system.** Whatever your concern or problem may be, your primary care doctor will either be able to either treat it or determine precisely when and where to send you for specialized help. In either case, you have the distinct advantage of a physician's expertise, and any trips through the medical "maze" will be less confusing for you... and less of a hassle.
- **Preventive healthcare.** Your primary care doctor can help you with disease prevention, as well as prompt intervention during any illness.
- **Continuity of care.** You and your doctor can develop and sustain an ongoing health partnership. He will get to know your concerns, and you won't have to repeat your history each time you fall ill or

need treatment. Your primary care doctor will know you as well as any chronic problems or potential troubles you may be facing. He will also be familiar with your family history.

- **One-stop shopping.** You can consult the same doctor for a variety of conditions, and often, he can treat both you and your family. Your family doctor can take you and your family through pregnancy, childbirth, and child care, thus instilling the concept of good health at an early age.

- **Lower cost and convenience.** Primary care doctors generally serve large populations of patients, so they encounter and become familiar with managing the most common medical maladies. They have been trained to diagnose and treat a wide range of conditions cost-effectively. And, in most cases, it's easier to gain access to a primary care doctor than a specialist, since general practices are usually geared to maximum efficiency.

Your primary care physician should be someone who will coordinate and oversee your overall medical care, referring you to a specialist only if needed. It is not usually a good idea to consult the "top" specialist for every problem; for example, rushing to a neurologist for a headache. Such a step can actually lead to your receiving poor, expensive care! Specialists sometimes order unnecessary tests (which can be expensive and painful) to rule out rare diseases (after all, they are specialists, and they cannot afford to overlook any possibility, however, remote it may be, when making a diagnosis).

On the other hand, a generalist who does not specialize in that particular field may also order unnecessary tests for fear of missing something. Thus, it is important that you find a primary care doctor who is confident enough to order the basic necessary tests but also knows when to refer you to a specialist for those more specific tests that he is not as qualified to render.

Using a Specialist as a Primary Care Doctor

Many patients prefer a general practitioner (also known as a family physician), a general physician, or an internist. However, there are definitely reasons to prefer a specialist. For example, a woman may prefer to see a gynecologist, and for your children you may choose to go to a pediatrician.

In addition, depending on the level of care you need to receive, a specialist may be a better bargain than a generalist. Although he or she may charge a little more per visit, he or she can home in on the problem more quickly and save time and money on unnecessary tests. For example, if you have had a history of gastrointestinal problems and continue to have them, a gastroenterologist may be you best source for a primary care doctor for the simple reason that if your problems persist, you would not need a referral (depending on your insurance) and the more experienced he is, the less equipment and tests he will perform on you, thus charging you less.

Being Nice Pays Off

Your doctor can be your best ally and advocate for medical discounts if you choose the right one. (See Chapter 16 for more details on getting discounts.) Befriend your doctor. Doctors, like almost all other professionals, will work harder for patients who are kind and reliable than those who are confrontational and difficult. It is a fact of life. Physicians are not obligated to expedite tests or ensure that a patient receives the best care, but you need to remember that physicians will treat kind, reliable patients, regardless of their income, race, or socioeconomic status. Your doctor will become your most important voice in times of distress or illness and will push harder for patients who have not been difficult. Doctors are not obligated to go above and beyond the call of duty, but often this is needed to get the best care.

Often a physician will be happy to write off a favorite patient's medical bill, if *asked*. Request a discount! Most patients who ask for a break on their bill will get some form of discount. Don't be shy. Invite your doctor out to play golf, offer him some basketball tickets, or simply bake your favorite brownies for him. This will prove to be one of the best investments in your future you could make, not to mention that it may save you money on your next medical bill!

Where to Find a Doctor

Find a doctor when you don't need one. This statement may seem paradoxical, but finding the right doctor when you are ill is much more difficult, because of the stress of the illness—as well as the pressure of time.

When you are beginning your search, your first step should be to ask your friends for recommendations. A good source of referrals can be nurses and other paramedical staff. If you have a friend who is a doctor, seek his advice as well. Local teaching hospitals are the best places to survey doctors. Nurses are always happy to help you choose a doctor and will not only recommend one who is competent, but one they like working with. To you, this translates into a doctor who has good a bedside manner.

The yellow pages can also serve as a useful source of possible names if you need to make a comprehensive list. You can phone the doctors on your list. Although it may appear unorthodox, "telephone shopping" can provide you with a lot of useful information about individual doctors' practice, including details of clinic timings, fees, qualifications, hospital affiliations, and special interests. You can learn a good deal about the doctor and his practice, even before you actually meet him, by merely telephoning and asking the right questions.

Be your own investigator. If you ask the right questions, you will get the answers you want, which will help you make the right decisions. If you are uncomfortable with the answers, there is probably a reason.

Already in a Healthcare Plan?

If you are already in a healthcare plan, your choices may be limited to doctors who participate in the plan. Be sure you have an accurate and updated list from your insurance provider of doctors within its network. Do all the research mentioned previously until you feel comfortable with at least three doctors on that list.

Most insurance companies require that you have a primary care doctor, i.e., a physician who can serve as the gatekeeper for your referrals, take care of basic medical needs, carry out regular checkups; and treat common illnesses.

Next, call the doctor and make sure he or she is accepting new patients. Unfortunately, a good doctor may not have room to add a new patient; however, be sure to ask him or her if a doctor can be recommended who is accepting new patients as well as your healthcare plan. By the time you get through your list, you make come across a doctor that is new to the area, new to the field, but has the confidence of at least two doctors on your list that were not accepting patients.

By using a referral from a doctor who is not accepting new patients, you might find a hidden gem. A good doctor will almost never recommend a "bad doctor" because his reputation is at stake, and news of a bad doctor can spread very fast throughout the medical community as well as the general public. A doctor who recommends a "bad doctor" will be questionable.

Check Your Doctor's Background

It's extremely important, once you have a list of potential doctors, to do some background research. Keep in mind that not every doctor has the same type of training and experience, even those within the same specialty, especially in today's advanced medical healthcare environment. In addition, no doctor will tell you outright whether he or she has been disciplined or had one or more malpractice judgments issued against him or her. The only way to find out is to ask or research the surgeon or physician yourself.

How can you research a doctor? The Internet is loaded with sites that claim to have information about doctors' credentials information; however, you want to make sure you get more than just a doctor's license number and contact information. For more comprehensive information, consider contacting the following sources.

- **Your local library.** More specifically, you can look up basic information about doctors in the *Directory of Medical Specialists*. This reference has up-to-date professional and biographic information on about 400,000 practicing physicians.
- **Your state medical board.** It should have a record of complaints or disciplinary actions taken against the doctor.
- **Your state department of insurance.** It's a good idea to check to see if the doctor has any complaints against him or her with this department, but remember that not all departments of insurance accept complaints.
- **The American Board of Medical Specialties (ABMS).** This nonprofit organization includes 24 medical specialty boards.
- **Medical society of the field of specialty.** There are many societies in the medical field. Try finding your intended physician or surgeon in one. The United States Medical Specialists Federation has a partial list of these societies listed at www.usmsf.us, as does the American Medical Association (AMA) at www.ama-assn.org/ama/pub/category/15378.html.
- **American Medical Association (AMA).** Unfortunately, this applies only if you are a member. The phone number is 312-464-5000. The same information can be found in "Physician Select" on the AMA website: http://webapps.ama-assn.org/doctorfinder/home.html?aps/amahg.htm.

Keep in mind that doctors are not required to join associations such as the AMA or other medical societies. In fact, more and more doctors are choosing not to due to the time and financial commitments with no guaranteed outcome. So do not let the lack of association membership be a deterrent for your decision.

Also, don't be afraid to ask health insurance plans and medical offices for information on their doctors' training and experience. They may have more information than you think.

The more research you conduct into a doctor's background, the more it will increase your chances of finding a healthcare provider who will fulfill your medical needs.

You may want to start your search by contacting your state medical board or by browsing online. Most state medical boards do not charge; however, most (if not all) offer only limited background information on doctors. The state medical boards or state medical licensure is usually located under the Department of Health in your state. They should have updated records of every doctor practicing legally as well as those practicing on a pending license.

A website that contains contact information for licensing physicians in 40 states and the District of Columbia is www.hospicepatients.org/check-physicians.html. The site information varies, but most of the ones listed should have at least the names of doctors they discipline on their website. Unfortunately, 10 states provide no information over the Internet about doctors disciplined by their licensing boards. They are Alaska, Arkansas, Delaware, Hawaii, Louisiana, Montana, New Mexico, North Dakota, South Dakota, and Wyoming; however, more and more states are starting to post comprehensive physician profiles. Another site that provides the same type of information is www.docboard.org.

The American Board of Medical Specialties (866-275-2267 or 866-ASK-ABMS) can tell you if the doctor is board certified. "Certified" means that the doctor has completed a training program in a specialty and has passed an exam (board) to assess his or her knowledge, skills, and experience to provide quality patient care in that specialty. Primary care doctors may also be certified as specialists. You can also check the website www.certifacts.org.

Another resource of physician background checking is through a private establishment; however, very few establishments (less than a handful) specialize in providing information relating to doctors' credentials. That's why it's important to find out how credible the company is and what type of doctor-related information it offers.

Doctors' Credentials

Just looking at a doctor's credentials does not guarantee that you will receive high-quality healthcare. While many of us tend to be overawed by a long list of alphabets behind the doctor's name, you need to remember that not all of them are legitimate degrees, and if they are, are you paying for the extra letters?

Some doctors without an M.D. call themselves "Doctor" to give the impression that they have an "M.D." or have been to medical school in the United States, when they have actually have not. Even graduates from small, understaffed Caribbean medical schools are awarded an "M.D.," so this can be deceiving. (Students at Caribbean medical schoold are universally those who were rejected by all the U.S. medical schools to which they applied.) Similarly, a DO (doctor of osteopathy) often could not matriculate in a U.S. medical school). This does not necessarily mean that such doctors are worse than a U.S. graduate who has an M.D. For example, someone who received a medical degree from another country may have gone through a different training program than a doctor educated in the United States. Some are more rigorous and some are less rigorous. Some have more of a "hands-on" program with less emphasis on the intricacies, such as the medical lingo. Other medical programs accept many students at once and others only a limited number.

The United States has certain standards that medical students from other countries must obtain in order to practice in the United States. If a doctor does not pass these tests, he or she may be granted only a "limited license" and have to take extra courses to bring him or her up to speed with U.S. practices. Some may not feel it is necessary to obtain these extra certification qualifications to practice general medicine, but be careful: some doctors may be practicing advanced medicine without the extra certification and have not yet been tested.

Many doctors use FACP (Medicine), FACS (Surgery), FACG (Gastroenterology), FRCP (U.K.), MRCP (U.K.), and other such abbreviations after their degree. These are often not educational qualifications but awards bestowed upon the physician for years of service, teaching, or membership. The most important qualification of your physician really is the quality of training he or she received *after* medical school. The locations of internship and residency, fellowships and advanced fellowship, and publications in clinical research can often mean more than where a doctor received his M.D. It is very important to know your doctor's educational and training background and check his credentials (see www.docinfo.org). After all, this is your health we are talking about!

If you are going to have surgery, check out the credentials of a surgeon by inquiring about him from those who know him or have been operated upon by him. This category includes other patients as well as colleagues of the surgeon. One good way of finding the ideal surgeon is to find out whom doctors go to when they need surgery for themselves or their families. The greatest compliment to a surgeon is paid when he is chosen by a doctor or his family.

The Castle Connolly guide at www.castleconnolly.com/index. cfm?dws=ey, as well as DrScore at www.drscore.com, are two websites that rate U.S. doctors. Many national ranking publications allow doctors to be paid in their listing in order to produce more revenue; however, the above-mentioned are two sources that are quite reputable and do not allow this to happen or online or in print. Castle Connelly is a physician-led research team that surveys physicians every year in order to identify the very best in every specialty for every kind of problem. DrScore surveys patients, giving them an opportunity to rate their doctor and the quality of service they have received. There are many other local surveys held in many other parts of the county similar to this one that can help you in your decision process. Just be sure, the surveys are done by the doctors/surgeons or even patients who have been to these doctors themselves and are confidential.

Following are some basic but important criteria to consider when seeking an experienced, well-trained physician or a good surgeon.

- If you are looking for a specialist, make sure he or she is board-certified in his/her respective field of specialty.
- Make sure no disciplinary actions have been instituted against the practitioner.
- Look closely at malpractice judgments and how many have been brought against the practitioner. (More than three is not good.)
- Find out if he or she is fellowship-trained in his or her specialty field. This is usually a good sign.
- The more hospital affiliations or membership affiliations the doctor has, the better.

- Check to see if the physician or surgeon has been practicing medicine for five years or more.
- If the doctor has teaching responsibilities at any hospitals or other medical institutions, it's a very good sign.
- Find out how much of the physician's practice focuses on the medical condition or surgery you are requesting.
- Find out if the physician/surgeon has received any awards or is involved in his/her community.
- Pay attention to what other people in the community say about the physician.

Decide What You Want and Need in a Doctor

Once you have a list of doctors who may meet your needs and have researched their backgrounds to make sure they have the expertise you are looking for, it's time for the next step. What makes a "good doctor" for you? Spend some time investigating what is most important to you in a doctor. A few ideas are listed below. Add your own to create a list that will help you choose a doctor who is right for you.

If your number one concern is that your doctor is highly rated by a consumer or other group, for example, you will want to find out who did the ratings and if the information is reliable. Who collected the information? Does the group judging the rankings have something to gain from rating doctors a certain way?

You may feel that your doctor needs to have experience with your condition(s). Research shows that doctors who have a lot of experience with a condition tend to have better success with it. If this is a major concern to you, your research should emphasize this.

A key point to keep in mind is that not all doctors have privileges at the hospital of your choice. Be sure to check if a doctor is permitted to practice at your hospital. Ask his office staff where he practices and double-check with the hospital to be sure he still has these privileges.

As explained before, you doctor should be in your plan for you to avoid major charges. However, keep in mind that doctors are so busy these days that they may not realize that they have been dropped by an insurance plan. Be sure to check with not only the staff but your insurance plan as well as their contract dates. You don't want to get into a situation where you love the doctor but a month later, he does not accept your insurance or your insurance does not accept him.

Schedule a Visit

The next step is to schedule a visit with your top choice. During that first visit you will learn a lot about just how easy it is to talk with the doctor. You will also find out how well the doctor might meet your medical needs. Ask yourself: Did the doctor. . .

- Give me a chance to ask questions?
- Really listen to my questions?
- Answer in terms I understood?
- Show respect for me?
- Ask me questions?
- Make me feel comfortable?
- Address the health problem(s) I came with?
- Ask me my preferences about various kinds of treatments?
- Spend enough time with me?

Trust your own reactions when deciding whether a certain doctor is the right one for you. But you also may want to give the relationship some time to develop. It will take more than one visit for you and your doctor to get to know each other.

Although some of these questions may be redundant, these are the ones to ask that will affect your bottom line and should almost definitely be considered if you want to save money on your medical bill:

- Is your doctor more concerned about your bottom line or his paycheck?
- Is the location of the doctor's clinic important? (In other words, How far do I have to drive? Is there parking?)
- What days/hours does the doctor see patients? Are the times convenient?
- Do I have to choose a doctor who is covered by my insurance plan?
- Is the doctor duly qualified and in which field? For example, a patient with a heart problem may prefer to see a cardiologist rather than a general physician.
- How far in advance do I have to make appointments?
- What is the length of an average visit?
- In case of an emergency, how fast can I see the doctor?
- Who takes care of patients after hours, i.e., when the doctor is on call or away?

- Does he actively listen to you (show interest in your overall health), explain the relevant facts, ask you questions, and answer your questions?
- Does he explain everything in "your language," including diagnosis, procedures, treatment, and what you can expect in the future, so you will understand?
- Does he give you valid reasons for treatment plans or tests ordered?
- Is he up to date with the relevant information?
- Is he open to discussion about alternative systems?
- Does he prescribe medication that you can afford, such as generics?
- Does he fit you in if you are really sick despite having a tight schedule?
- Does he refer you to various sources (e.g., books, journals, the Internet) to clarify information?
- Does he refer you to an appropriate specialist when required?
- Does he refer you to other support services or self-help groups?
- Does he or his staff phone back when additional information or test results are obtained?
- Does he give adequate consultation time?
- Does the doctor have hospital privileges at a respected medical institution?

Some things that are signs of a bad doctor are that he or she:
- Does not value your time and makes you wait interminably on a routine basis
- Is more interested in treating your reports than in treating you
- Does not spend enough time with you or explain your treatment so that you understand
- Seems to be too busy and rushed all the time
- Orders tests whether or not they are needed
- Does not explain your options to you
- Discourages questions or refuses to answer them
- Promises too much
- Makes remarks such as "I'll look into my crystal ball" or "that's my secret"
- Discourages second opinions

If you are searching for a surgeon, the best place to begin your search is to ask your primary care doctor. To start with, your doctor knows you and your situation better than any other physician. Since most doctors are aware of the accomplishments of "superspecialists" who practice at large university hospitals or research-based facilities, your doctor can help you identify the experts. If you can find a book or article relating to your problem, the author (if he is a doctor) is likely to be a good choice. The other option is to find the name of a doctor or the head of a clinic or department who is actively publishing medical research in this field. This doctor (or the head of the clinic) is likely to be an authority in the subject and will be well informed of the latest advances in the field.

If you are not satisfied with the answers to the proceeding questions, discuss your concerns with your doctor. If you are still not satisfied even after this discussion, you should consider looking for another doctor.

When You Have to Change Doctors

Changing doctors is never easy, because over a period of time you do build up a personal relationship with your doctor. However, you should consider changing doctors if you strongly feel that:

- **The doctor is incompetent.** For example, he has ignored obvious symptoms, missed a diagnosis, prescribed the wrong drug, or can't get to the bottom of your problem.
- **The doctor does not communicate with you effectively.** His explanations are short and not easily understood, and he does not give you time to ask questions. The doctor does not pay attention to your needs and concerns.
- **You have lost confidence in the doctor's skill and ability.**
- **You find the doctor is too inconsiderate.** For example, he consistently makes you wait a long time for an appointment, fails to return your phone calls, or does not provide clinic time during evening or weekend hours.
- **The doctor is too expensive**.

In the final analysis, remember that the most reliable test for a doctor's suitability for you is your own gut instinct—if you don't feel comfortable with your doctor, you should not hire him as your doctor. Would you leave a stranger alone in your house? Chances are you would not. On the other hand, if you have faith in his abilities and can trust that he will do his best for you, you are likely to get excellent medical care!

Unfortunately, you may have only one option when it comes to health insurance when it limits your medical choices. This may happen if some of the more established doctors do not choose to accept your health insurance due to the constraints on their reimbursement. You may find that these constraints are straining your doctor's ability to take care of your healthcare needs. In this case, you need to decide if you should find other means of obtaining healthcare coverage, rather than changing doctors. This is where your "partnership" with your doctor may come into play.

If your doctor suddenly drops your insurance, make sure you find out from him or his staff. You may find that your insurance policy has changed so dramatically that it may be worth the investment of purchasing a new insurance policy. Have a candid conversation with someone who deals with health insurance on a daily basis, such as the billing manager or the physician. Ask what insurance they would recommend and why. You may uncover some details that will affect you in the future if they have not already affected your bottom line.

If your doctor is retiring, ask him to recommend a doctor who accepts your insurance and be sure the retiring doctor reviews your chart with the recommended doctor. Be sure the retiring doctor has a close enough relationship with the recommended doctor that the current he could still have say in your treatment if necessary. If the recommended doctor has time, it may be wise to set up an appointment with both together. Again, if you are uncomfortable with the new doctor who is recommended, chances are your instincts are right. You may have to ask around for a "good" doctor.

However, do not get into the habit of switching doctors, because your initial visit will cost about three times more than your following visits. Every time you have an initial visit, you will pay an initial fee as well as its being more time consuming, as you will be required to fill out paperwork.

Best advice: When you find a doctor you like, stick with him and build upon that relationship. It will save you a lot of time, money, and headaches. Just be sure you invest time in the initial background research of your doctor. You will be glad you did!

CHAPTER 2

THE DOCTOR VISIT

NO ONE LIKES TO GET SICK, and, as a logical extension, most of us don't like going to the doctor. However, one should never forget that the doctor-patient relationship is unique; it is a relationship in which you confide fully in your doctor and entrust him with your life. You must learn to work with your doctor as a partner. Research has shown that patients who have a good relationship with their doctor tend to be more satisfied with their care—and to have better results. This chapter will provide you with some basic tips on how to foster a solid partnership with your doctor while getting the most out of your doctor visit.

Respect Your Doctor and the Staff

Respect is the best way to nurture the relationship with your doctor, and most doctors recognize this, even if they are having a bad day. It is amazing how many patients forget to say "thank you" to their doctor when they get better. Keep in mind, your doctor deals with droves of patients with complaints all day long and would be delighted to hear a patient appreciate his efforts. This simple expression of gratitude will help the doctor to remember you as a person, rather than as just another case. He is likely to then treat you as a special patient, and getting VIP attention from him will help improve your medical care a good deal.

My internist is one of the busiest doctors in the D.C. area. Patients will wait weeks to schedule an appointment with him. He is not accepting any new patients because his schedule is so packed; however, he always makes room for me. I have been a patient of his for over 10 years. I've heard him describe me as a sweet elderly lady with three grandchildren who are all graduating from college and live in different states. The other day, one of my grandchildren was visiting from out of town and suddenly came down with the flu. I called my doctor's office the next day to try to get an appointment, but his receptionist informed me that he was booked solid that day. Later the same day, when he found out that I had called to try to book an appointment, he called me back and squeezed my grandchild into his schedule first thing the next day. My good relationship with my doctor definitely proved to be a valuable asset to me and my family.

—Melissa Jones, age 72

As in a marriage, the doctor-patient relationship depends on good communication and trust built up over time, and it is definitely worth spending the time and taking the trouble to maintain a beneficial relationship.

Remember that the doctor's staff plays a key role in your medical care, and you need to learn how the clinic functions. It's very helpful to build up a rapport with a special staff member (who may be a receptionist, a nurse, or an assistant), and this can prove to be very useful when you need to talk to the doctor on a priority basis. A small thank-you gift for the staff can help ensure that you get personalized attention.

Do Your Homework

Your visits to the doctor may be expensive, despite the fact that the actual time you get to spend with your doctor is very short. Many doctors have perfected the technique of flying into the examination room, shooting off questions, and rattling off advice. And, before you know it, you're shoved out the door, worrying about those crucial matters you forgot to ask and the directions you forgot to write down. Do your homework thoroughly before visiting the doctor.

In order to make the best use of your doctor's time, you need to prepare for your visit. A well-organized patient not only makes efficient use of the doctor's time but is also likely to get better medical care, as he is helping the doctor a great deal in making an accurate diagnosis. A conscientious patient makes sure that he has all his medical records with him (and takes along copies of all labs, tests, screenings, and so on from previous doctors), as well as the vital questions to which he needs answers (preferably in writing).

Patients who value the doctor's time will do their best to get answers to their queries by tapping external sources such as books, libraries, and the Internet before going to the doctor's clinic. This procedure will allow them and their doctor to focus on what is important to them, so that they can make the best use of the limited quality time that they have with the doctor.

Remember to inform your doctor about all the symptoms you have noted. List them in chronological order, starting from the time when you first noted that something was amiss. It's extremely useful to record the factors that make your symptoms better and those that make them worse. This information provides very useful medical clues. Also, let your doctor know what remedies you have tried earlier and whether they helped or not. If you have previously consulted another doctor or have undergone relevant tests, please share this information with your present doctor.

It's helpful to prepare a short one-page summary of your medical history; not only does this summary help the doctor, but it will also ensure that you do not forget to convey to him information that could be vitally important in your treatment. Computer programs are available that can help you record and organize your medical history, as well as those of your family members. Make a list of all the medications you are taking, both prescription and nonprescription. As an alternative, you can collect all your medicines in a brown paper bag and show them to your doctor. In addition, list all the specialists you are consulting for specific disorders or conditions.

Not everyone can remember his or her specialists and what each specialist specializes in, so instead of trying to remember, write it all down. This will help you organize your thoughts and remember your questions. These written checklists should be carried with you during every visit. Normally, you can think up a wide range of questions to ask the doctor, but as a result of the stress generated by the consultation you invariably forget most of them and waste your money. To prevent this from happening, write down all the questions you need to ask in order of priority. It is also helpful to write down the doctor's answers. Studies have shown that patients forget about 50 percent of what the doctor tells them during a visit.

Your doctor also stands to benefit because you need not pester him with your queries arepeatedly, thus strengthening your relationship. Thus you will be more efficient with your time with your doctor, and save yourself money. Similar to an attorney, a doctor can bill every 15 minutes as well as for every symptom you mention as a different alignment. By making sure you arrive at your appointment with a list of questions, you'll have all your questions answered.

Question the office about billing procedures. It is not unusual to request an itemized bill at the time of the initial visit. Make sure your doctor does not leave until all questions are answered. You may also want to request a discount on the "above insurance" balance that will become due at the initial consultation. In other words, after your insurance is paid, you may want to ask for a discount on the remaining amount that you are expected to pay.

Ask for a Diagnosis

Ultimately, you want to know what the diagnosis is, so do not shirk from asking your doctor what he thinks is wrong with you. Surprisingly, many doctors are reluctant to give a name to a patient's problems, so that if you do not ask specifically, you may not get an answer. If you do not agree with the doctor's diagnosis, tell him so, because if you do not agree with it, you are unlikely to follow his advice and treatment.

Often, your doctor may reply he does not know the diagnosis as yet. This response does not indicate that he is an incompetent physician; it may simply mean that you have a difficult problem, for which more tests are needed. It might also mean that your doctor would like to "wait and watch" to see how the problem evolves or that he may need to refer you for a second opinion.

Ask your doctor to explain your diagnosis and how it might affect you and your family. Useful questions include:

- What is the diagnosis? Find out the complete medical name—and what it means in plain English!
- What is my prognosis (outlook for the future)?
- What changes, if any, will I need to make in my daily life?
- Is there a chance that someone else in my family might get the same condition?
- Will I need special help at home for my condition? If so, what type of help?

Again, you must tell him everything you know, think, and feel about your problem if you want an accurate diagnosis and the best treatment plan for the smallest amount of money. There is no need to be shy or embarrassed about sensitive subjects such as sexual problems or sexually transmitted diseases. The more open you are, the less of a mystery your diagnosis will become and the fewer tests may be ordered, meaning less money out of your pocket.

Do not hesitate to share your thoughts with your doctor. If you think that what he is recommending does not make sense, say so and specify your reasons. If you do not, your doctor will assume that you are not interested in a full explanation of your illness and its treatment.

You are entitled to raise all relevant questions and seek satisfactory answers to them. If you cannot understand your doctor's explanations, politely ask him to repeat everything in simpler language. Ask him to show you illustrations; also, ask for written material or website URLs that may explain the medical issue(s) in greater detail so that you can study them later at your leisure.

Try to schedule your next visit at the end of the consultation. If the succeeding question-and-answer session is something that can be managed on the telephone, try to do so. You could save both time and money by avoiding an unnecessary follow-up visit to the doctor's clinic.

Try to find a friend or relative to accompany you to the consultation, as his or her presence can be very useful. He or she can help reduce your anxiety, give you courage to ask the relevant questions, and help you interpret the doctor's statements. As mentioned earlier, do not hesitate to ask ques-

---

How To Make Your Doctor's Receptionist Think You're Terrific

If you're well organized and prepared when you phone or visit your doctor's clinic, you'll win the respect and the doctor and appreciation of the receptionist and staff, which will make him that much more helpful in helping you get the best medical care. For example, when you telephone with regard to a medical problem, the following guidelines can be very useful:

- Introduce yourself. State briefly (in one sentence) why you're calling. ("I've had fever of 101° for three days, and I was wondering if there's something else I should be doing about it apart from taking Tylenol"). If you don't think your problem is serious enough to merit a visit to the doctor, say so.
- Be prepared to answer the following questions: What are the specific symptoms? When (what day/time) did the symptoms start? What have you done for relief, if anything? (Refer to your notes for the names of any prescribed or over-the-counter medication you may have taken.) What is the main cause of your anxiety? How would you like to be helped?
- Keep a pencil or pen and paper handy to take notes.

tions (and more questions); never mind how many other patients are waiting in the doctor's clinic or how stupid the questions may seem to you. When you are with the doctor, his only focus of interest should be you, and it's his job to provide answers. Be courteous but assertive while asking questions and obtaining information, but don't turn aggressive or antagonistic. Listen carefully to what your doctor says, and in case of doubt or ambiguity, do not leave till they have been dispelled.

If you disagree on a treatment option, you should speak to him about it immediately. Let me point out that there's a right way of approaching your doctor and a wrong way. Often, if you can put across your feelings and apprehensions in the right way, you can get your doctor to help you. Explain your needs to your physician in a polite way, without any belligerence or hostility. Remember that you are both on the same side—yours!

Waiting for the Doctor

The most common complaint of patients is that they are made to wait for ages before the doctor can see them. Some patients seem to believe that the longer they have to wait outside the doctor's clinic, the better he must be, since he has so many patients clamoring for his attention. This is simply not true. No matter how hard pressed a doctor may be, he can always space out his appointments so that you never have to wait for more than an hour to see him. Some exceptions are specialists who deal with emergency situations in which the operating room relies solely on their expertise.

Be patient. You may want to alert the staff as to your expected wait time so they can adjust the appointment times. Remember, in most cases, it is the staff who scheduled you, not the doctor. If you are waiting more that thirty minutes and the clinic staff is not courteous enough to provide an explanation and, if needed, an alternate appointment, you should complain to the hospital or office manager, who will rectify matters.

In order to ensure that you don't lose your patience while waiting in the clinic, it would be a prudent idea to carry a paperback novel or a portable CD player. Nowadays, many doctors keep educational leaflets and brochures in their clinics, and you could read these and thus use your waiting time constructively.

In addition, keep this as a bargaining chip for a time when you might be late due to an unforeseen circumstance such as a flat tire, traffic, or children, and don't get upset.

Help Your Doctor Stay Organized—and Save

Make sure you carry photocopies of all your medical records and tests the day you get them. They are free and it will save you time in case you need a second opinion etc. Waiting until "you need them" will only cost more and delay your treatment because you will have to pay extra for your primary doctor to send them, but first, the staff may have to find these records. You can give them to the doctor copies for his files, if needed—but keep your originals with you—they are your property. Also, make sure that you have clearly understood the contents of your medical records so that you can explain the details to another doctor if needed.

Please remember that in over 80 percent of cases, you can be diagnosed on your medical history and what you tell your doctor. This should emphasize the importance of being able to talk to your doctor intelligently. While the capability of absorbing the relevant details of an individual's medical

---

Certain categories of patients can be particularly irksome or tiresome. For instance, doctors dislike patients who:

- Expect to be treated on a priority basis
- Cancel appointments constantly or cancel without calling
- Are always late
- Waste time needlessly
- Ask the same questions endlessly
- Think they know all the answers
- Do not value the doctor's privacy or personal time
- Do not follow instructions
- Change doctors all the time
- Don't pay their fees on time
- Cannot explain exactly what's bothering them
- Answer questions dishonestly
- Do not volunteer any important information that the doctor may not specifically ask about, including family history
- Do not let the doctor know if they cannot follow his directions and do not specify the reasons why
- Do not take medications as directed, strictly adhering to the dose schedule
- Do not express their dissatisfaction in a courteous manner

history is one of the key skills of a competent physician, being able to provide a lucid history is a key skill on the part of a good patient and makes for a less expensive visit.

In this context, a useful aide-mémoire includes the following details:

Site: Location (e.g., pain is in the chest and then spreads to the left arm).

Quantity: Bringing up a cupful of sputum when coughing.

Quality: It feels like an elephant is sitting on my chest!

Setting: I usually develop such aches after fighting with my husband.

Aggravating factors: Stomachache becomes worse after eating.

Alleviating factors: Breathlessness becomes better after resting.

Sample Worksheet

Site: _____

Quantity: _____

Setting: _____

Aggravating factors: _____

Alleviating factors: _____

If you remember to categorize all your problems systematically, not only will you make better use of your time with your doctor but you can also help him arrive at a correct diagnosis more quickly. By providing relevant information about your health status, both past and present, you can help your doctor help you. The following aspects need to be highlighted:

- Your medical history (including instances of surgery and hospitalization)
- Your family's medical history
- Allergies you are prone to
- Medications you have taken (and are still taking)
- Your daily routine

• Your work schedule
• Pressures you have been subject to (and are still subject to)

No one knows you better than yourself, so stay organized and be as honest and pleasant as possible with your doctor. Because of this, your doctor will not only be better able to monitor your health, he will want to help you, because he is vested not only as your physician, but as a friend.

Are You Doing the Doctor's Job?

A concerned doctor will organize his or her clinic and its functioning so as to minimize your visits and save you money—for example; blood samples can be collected in the clinic itself and forwarded to a reliable laboratory, so that you don't need to go there yourself. Similarly, many obstetricians do ultrasound scans in their clinic, so that patients need not run around from one place to another. It is often less expensive to have a minimally invasive procedure, such as a colonoscopy, done at an ambulatory surgical center than it is to have it done at a hospital. The downside is less monitoring and fewer support staff if something goes wrong, but if you are in good health, this is often a less expensive choice.

On the other hand, be sure you help your doctor and his staff stay organized and let them know of any updates or changes in your insurance. This is the patient's responsibility. The doctor and his staff are busy with many patients with many different insurance plans. The one thing you do not want is to find out that your bill was not paid due to misinformation. This can cost you and the physician not only monetarily but can be extremely untimely, adding agitation to the staff and the physician, thus straining your relationship.

If you feel you are doing all the work and getting no help, express this to your doctor. He or she may not realize what his or she doing because he or she is so busy, but communicating this might help him or her realize how his or her lack of administrative help is affecting your relationship. The doctor might then talk with his staff to see how they can accommodate you, within reason, and lend you some guidance if the office is too busy. Unfortunately, not all relationships work out, and some doctors are unwilling to accommodate patients for one reason or another. If you are unhappy with the explanation and your doctor is unwilling to help make the process easier, be prepared to begin the hunt for another primary care physician.

Your Doctor and the Phone

Today, many physicians make themselves, an assistant, or another staff member available to their patients over the phone. Previsit questions and routine follow-up on the phone can save you—and your doctor—both time and money. Before making a call, you need to ascertain relevant information in advance:

- When is the best time to call?
- What is the doctor's rule for returning calls?
- Whom should you speak with (e.g., assistant or nurse) if the doctor can't come to the phone?
- What is the phone number for emergency calls or for calls when the office is closed?
- Whom can you call if your doctor is out of town?

When you reach your doctor or his assistant over the phone, be prepared to:

- Identify yourself.
- Get to the core problem, especially if you've phoned after hours. (Have someone else call the doctor for you if you are unable to talk.)
- Define your problems and symptoms accurately but swiftly. Write them down and keep them near the telephone so you can report them quickly and completely.
- Report results of self-tests and other symptoms you have been keeping track of, such as a temperature of 101°F for two days, diarrhea that has lasted for 48 hours, and so on.
- Ask the doctor what you should do, and write down his instructions carefully. Ask the doctor to spell out any word if you are unsure about it.
- Ask if and when you should call back, or if you should come to the clinic.
- Ascertain what complications could occur that might require you to hurry to the emergency room.
- Don't forget to thank the doctor for talking to you on the telephone!

Sometimes, you may have to call a doctor when the clinic is closed. Remember, when you call a doctor after hours, he is trying to help you solve your immediate problem, not provide advice about your entire medical situation. Try to be specific in your complaint; you should know what medications you are currently taking and which of them has proved successful in the past. If you are not happy with the physician's advice, go to a 24-hour outpatient clinic and resort to an emergency room only if you feel you have a life-threatening emergency. The emergency room is extremely expensive!

When you plan a visit to the clinic, the following points shouild be kept in mind.

- Make sure you fix an appointment. Try to schedule it well in advance and call beforehand to confirm it.
- Try to reach the clinic on time, since the doctor's time (and yours!) is precious.
- Make sure you have brought along all your records and documents.
- Try to cooperate with the staff. For example, if the doctor is running late, rather than pepper the staff with questions read a book or magazine while waiting.
- Try to learn the names of the staff members. If you treat them like VIPs, you'll be treated like one as well!

If you are lucky, the staff member may be able to locate the physician and present the information directly to the physician. If you have a good relationship with your doctor, the physician may call in the necessary drug information to your local pharmacy if he is familiar with your condition and medical background without you having to waste time and money for an unnecessary appointment.

Conclusion

By following these simple steps, you will not only gain the respect of the doctor and his staff, but you may also save a ton of money! Just be sure to be courteous when giving or receiving information. Everybody is human, even doctors, which means that they have good days and bad days. Some doctors wear their days on their sleeves, others are better at hiding it, but no matter what type of day you or your doctor are having, be sure that when he sees you, the experience is pleasant.

Give information:
- Don't wait to be asked.
- You know important things about your symptoms and your health history.
- Tell your doctor what you think he or she needs to know.
- It is important to tell your doctor personal information—even if it makes you feel embarrassed or uncomfortable.
- Bring a "health history" list with you (and keep it up to date).
- You can use the form provided in this guide. You might want to make a copy of the form for each member of your family.
- Always bring any medicines you are taking or a list of those medicines (including when and how often you take them).
- Talk about any allergies or reactions you have had to your medicines.
- Tell your doctor about any natural or alternative medicines or treatments.
- Bring other medical information, such as x-ray films, test results, and medical records.

Get information:
- Ask questions. If you don't, your doctor may think you understand everything that was said.
- Write down your questions before your visit. List the most important ones first to make sure they get asked and answered
- You might want to bring someone along to help you ask questions.
- This person can also help you understand and/or remember the answers.
- Ask your doctor to draw a picture if that might help explain something.
- Take notes.
- Some doctors do not mind if you bring a tape recorder to help you remember things. But always ask first.
- Let your doctor know if you need more time. If there is not time that day, perhaps you can speak to a nurse or physician assistant on staff. Or ask if you can call later to speak with someone.

Take information home:
- Ask for written instructions.
- Your doctor also may have brochures and audio and videotapes that can help you. If not, ask how you can get such materials.
- Once you leave the doctor's office, follow up.
- If you have questions, call.
- If your symptoms get worse, or if you have problems with your medicine, call your doctor.
- If you had tests sone and do not hear from your doctor, call for your test results.
- If your doctor said you need to have certain tests, make appointments at the lab or other offices to get them done.
- If your doctor said you should see a specialist, make an appointment.

CHAPTER 3

SECOND OPINIONS

AT PRESENT, GETTING A SECOND OPINION has become a common practice among doctors, which is why family physicians often consult with specialists and specialists, in turn, consult other specialists. If the process is misused, the patient may pay for it in the end; however, if you have a close relationship with your physician, and the physician is concerned about your health, the physician will have no problem being frank with you and referring you to someone who is more qualified to deal with your health issue instead of performing an overabundance of tests and consulting with no other physicians, including a specialist who is more qualified to identify the health issue.

It is not a bad indication if a doctor refers you to a specialist or a second opinion; in fact, it may be just the opposite. A second opinion proves very useful for patients afflicted with rare or complex problems. Unfortunately, some doctors tend to refer patients unnecessarily to other members of their "fraternity." Also, doctors will often cross-refer patients to each other for personal financial gain. In hospitals, especially, specialist consultation is often automatic and mandatory, and this process is inevitably overused, causing the patient's bill to shoot up! Thus, a hospitalized patient should ask the family physician (who should act as your medical manager) to intervene if the number of specialists involved in the treatment seems excessive.

It may be difficult to get an unbiased opinion from a second doctor who is a member of the staff in the same hospital as your doctor. If at all possible, you should consult an independent doctor in another hospital for a second opinion. Most medical insurance policies that cover consultation fees will pay for this.

If two different doctors happen to reach the same conclusion, at least you know you are on the right track! However, don't always assume that just because the opinions of both doctors are identical, you are safe. For example, if you have angina and you consult a cardiac surgeon, there is a high likelihood that he will advise you to undergo bypass surgery. A second cardiac surgeon is also likely to recommend the same; after all, it's just simple financial common sense from the surgeons' viewpoint! Therefore, getting a second opinion from a nonsurgical specialist (in this case, a cardiologist) can be helpful in preventing unnecessary surgery and costs.

When to Get a Second Opinion

It seems that more and more people will shop around for a car, house, even an outfit for a special event, and less time on investigating a recent diagnosis on a severe condition or terminal illness and do not get a second opinion.

In some cases, a second opinion can mean the difference between life and death, or just a boost of confidence that you and your doctor have made the correct decision regarding a treatment. Imagine having a lung, kidney, breast, or prostate removed, only to find out later that you were misdiagnosed. So, before getting treatment, get a second opinion! Getting a second opinion allows you not only to confirm the diagnosis but also to get a different perspective on your treatment options. Some doctors are more conservative and others more aggressive. By getting a second opinion, you get to hear *all* of your options.

It is also possible that another doctor might come up with a completely different and more promising option—one that your first doctor didn't think of or didn't know about. Following are some circumstances that may warrant a second opinion:

- When surgery is recommended. Keep in mind that about 80 percent of all surgery is elective (i.e., performed on a nonemergency basis and surgery is an expensive alternative).
- When the diagnosis reveals a rare, potentially fatal, or disabling disease. The original diagnosis could be incorrect and may need to be revised. Or, even if it is correct, there may be new or experimental treatments available at an institution specializing in the treatment of such a disease.
- When your symptoms persist unrelieved and the doctor can provide no satisfactory explanation for them.
- When the risks and benefits of the proposed procedures are not satisfactorily explained. The patient has a right to know the details

about risks and the cost involved and the potential benefits of any
procedure, test or surgery. It is preferable to get the relevant details
in writing, so that you can digest them at leisure.

- When the diagnostic procedures seem unnecessarily complex or
  expensive, or both. Some doctors are prone to making excessive use
  of technology in borderline situations, either due to insecurity or to
  protect themselves against malpractice litigation.
- When the patient lacks confidence in the doctor's ability to do all
  that can reasonably be done. Effective treatment demands trust, and
  a lack of trust is as valid a reason as any other for getting a second
  opinion or even another primary care doctor.

Again, I cannot emphasize how important it is to find the right doctor
for you from the beginning. Bottom line is if you get to the point where
you lack the confidence in your doctor as described above, you might make
the wrong decision in a desperate situation, thus costing you more in time,
tests, etc. Take your time to find a doctor you trust when you do not need
one!

Sources of Second Opinions

A great source of second opinions is doctors who practice in public/teach-
ing hospitals. The staff members here are basically academicians. Since they
teach medical students and residents, they are usually well read and well
informed. Moreover, since they do not have a financial stake in providing
you with advice, their information is likely to be reliable and accurate. It is
not uncommon to have to wait for a long period of time to see these doctors, but in the end, it is well worth the wait!

It is also possible to get a second opinion from a doctor who practices
alternative medicine, for example, homoeopathy. Such an opinion will provide a completely different perspective of looking at a problem, and you
may prefer this alternative.

You should also keep in mind that there are other ways of getting a second opinion apart from going to another doctor such as health books and
encyclopedias as the Internet! For example, you can "Ask the Doctor" at
www.flora.org/ask-doctor/, a free site that forwards your medical queries
to specialists from all over the world, who then give their respective opinions on your problem. You may also want to tap into newer resources such

as the National Institutes of Health at www.nih.gov. There are more sources to help you research your healthcare options mentioned later in this chapter. The following paragraphs will help you determine the legitimacy of your second opinion and other added tests that might warrant a more accurate diagnosis.

If it happens that your second opinion disagrees with the first, it's definitely worthwhile to get a family physician (preferably one who has no vested interest in the matter) to advise you. It would also be prudent to discuss the differences in the two opinions with the concerned doctors, so that they can explain and justify the reasons for the discrepancies in their diagnoses or plan of treatment.

Don't Be Taken for a Ride

A sure sign that your "second opinion" is taking advantage of you is if a doctor orders tests immediately instead of examining you, and listening to what you have to say. Listening works both ways: patient to doctor and doctor to patient. However, keep in mind that it is not uncommon for a doctor to reorder a test due to the fact that he may feel the initial doctor may have missed something after having an extensive conversation with you about the problem. If the test reorders is "targeted" to the problem mentioned that is OK, but if you find a doctor is reordering every test, even ones that do not seem to be related to the health problem, be sure to question him immediately. If you are not satisfied with the response, find another doctor.

Here is a general checklist of questions you should ask your doctor when a test is recommended:

- Why is the test being ordered?
- Is it to screen for a disease that has no symptoms, such as diabetes?
- Is it because the doctor is pretty certain about a diagnosis but needs the test to confirm it?
- Is it because the doctor is really puzzled about the diagnosis and is trying to rule out as many possibilities as possible?
- How definitive is the test?
- Is it the "gold standard" for making the diagnosis?
- Will it reveal for sure that a condition is present or not, or must it be repeated or followed by more sophisticated tests?
- What precisely will the doctor be looking for in the results of these tests?

- What does he hope to learn from the tests?
- How accurate are they?

You can help improve the accuracy of certain tests by taking simple steps beforehand. Therefore, ask your doctor if you need to take any precautions before the test; for example, before a Pap smear, avoid douching, wearing a tampon or using birth control foams or jellies for five days before the test and avoid sex for two days before the test. Other tests require special preparations, and you must check that they have been carried out, to make sure the results are reliable. For example, certain x-rays, such as barium enemas and intravenous pyelograms, require a laxative before the x-ray. Not doing the preparation properly can lead to inadequate results, requiring a repeat preparation, a repeat x-ray, and a repeat bill. Colonoscopies require a "prep" 12 to 24 hours before the procedure is preformed as well as a clear liquid diet to clean out the system. Any material may interfere with the ability to view the wall of the colon. If the prep is done incorrectly the exam may have to be repeated. You may also want to check on the types of prep because some may be more tolerable to you than others.

Unfortunately, not all relationships work out. If worse comes to worse, be prepared to begin the hunt for another primary care physician.

Ask these questions before going into a test:

- Will there be any pain?
- What are the side effects?
- What are the risks? (Many common tests do not involve any risks at all. Invasive tests, that is, those that entail introducing instruments (such as endoscopes) or chemicals (such as barium) into the body, generally, involve some risks, which may include infection, allergic reaction, or injury to an internal organ. Sometimes, a test may lead to complications which are more dangerous than the benefit to be derived from the test results. While this is usually not the case, you need to consider the risk-benefit ratio of all tests, especially expensive and invasive ones.)
- Is this the best test for your problem?
- What is the risk of not having the test done, and what are the alternatives?
- How will the result of the test change the course of your treatment? (This is the single most important question you must ask.

And if the answer is that it really won't, then maybe you don't need the test at all.)

Remember that medical tests can be very helpful in pinpointing your problem, but they need to be used wisely and well and choosing the right doctor, as well as a solid second opinion can assure that this is being done. After you have received your "second opinion" and taken the appropriate tests to warrant an accurate diagnosis, you can then go over possible treatments with your doctor(s) and be confident in your doctor(s) are looking out for your best interest.

Choosing a Treatment

The decision-making process is different for each patient and depends on individual situations and requirements. Some patients may opt for expensive, high-tech treatment, while others in the same situation may prefer to wait and watch.

Each of us has a different personal decision-making style. It is for you to choose which one of the following best fits your own personal style for making medical decisions:

- You may prefer to make the final selection of your treatment after seriously considering your doctor's opinion.
- Others may prefer that the doctor make the final decision with regard to which treatment should be resorted to, after seriously considering your opinion.
- Some may prefer to make the final selection about which treatment they will receive on their own.
- And although I do not recommend this, but others, especially the elderly prefer to leave all decisions regarding treatment to their doctor.

It is imperative that you find a doctor who respects and understands your personal decision-making style. The reason being is that is throughout your treatment, your options may change and so will your priorities. Try to be as realistic and open-minded as possible. While the final outcome will always remain unknown at the time of making decisions, if you take the time and the trouble to make your own decisions, at least you will have the satisfaction of knowing that you tried your best!

Your first step to take would be to find out what kinds of treatment are available. You'll often find that a variety of treatment options exist, for instance:

• Medical therapy
• Surgery
• Physiotherapy
• Radiation therapy (for some cancers)
• Waiting and watching (also called "masterful inactivity")

Your doctor will be able to make several recommendations about treatment. A second opinion might help the doctor uncover other treatments he may not have thought of in the past or help him make a decision on the best treatment for you. If your doctor tells you that there is no beneficial treatment, think again! Maybe there is? For example, sometimes tumors are deemed inoperable by one surgeon but are found operable by another. Sometimes a closer examination of a case could change the diagnosis from one kind of cancer to another, more treatable type. Sometimes another doctor will know of a promising treatment that the first one didn't know about. All of these things have happened and continue to happen.

Be sure to pay attention and listen to your doctor. If he is using words such as "almost," "possible," "probably," "maybe," "chances," "unlikely," etc. you should, most definitely, get a second opinion. For instance, if your doctor says, "Your tumor is *probably* inoperable, and the *chances* of removing all of the cancer are *unlikely*," get a second opinion. Especially if your doctor suggests a treatment that simply sounds "off the wall" to you, get a second opinion or ask him to explain it further so you understand it better. For instance, if your doctor says "All the cancer in your left lobe of your lung is gone, but I think we should remove that lung anyway," get a second opinion. Conversely, if your doctor suggests "waiting" to see what happens, get a second opinion immediately. Waiting may give a disease like cancer the opportunity to spread and if you wait too long, it may be too late.

If you live in a rural area and/or get treatment at a small hospital, it may be beneficial to get a second opinion from a doctor at a major hospital or from a hospital that specializes in treating the disease you may have; you may even find a totally different diagnosis. Not all small rural hospitals are incompetent, in fact, some of the best doctors may prefer smaller hospitals and have affiliation or contacts in the bigger hospitals, but typically, the

New Technology in Medicine and Your Doctor

It is very easy (and very tempting) to misuse medical technology. For example, MRI (magnetic resonance imaging) scanners are the latest advance in technology, and these machines can undoubtedly provide very useful information about the human body! Machines such as MRI scanners are very expensive and need to be used for at least 10 scans a day to be cost-effective. Private hospitals buy them because they represent the "latest technology" and are in vogue. Unfortunately, in some rural areas, there are not enough patients to satisfy the 10 scans a day needed to break even. As a result, many patients are subjected to unnecessary scans, simply to keep the machines financially viable. Paradoxically, patients also pressurize doctors to misuse the new technology. Many of them go "doctor shopping" and demand that the latest whole-body scan be done to prove that they are healthy.

You need to be aware of the following inappropriate uses of medical technology.

- **Excessive use of technology, even when it is not required.** A prime example is an ultrasound scanning during pregnancy. While no one will dispute the fact that ultrasound scanning provides an extremely useful window to the fetus and can yield invaluable information, "cosmetic" ultrasound scans to provide "pictures" for the baby's first album are inappropriate and costly.
- **Unethical use of technology.** While prenatal diagnosis (using ultrasound scanning) has been a very important tool for reducing the risk of birth defects, it can also be used inappropriately, especially when it is misused for fetal sex selection by performing female feticide.
- **Use of technology that is not suitable for a particular patient.** An example of this would be advising IVF (in vitro fertilization) for all infertile patients, just because the equipment and expertise are available and the procedure is technically feasible. However, for most infertile patients, many simpler treatment options are available, which should be fully explored before considering IVF.

New Technology in Medicine and Your Doctor (Continued)

- **Misuse of technology by unqualified persons.** A common example is the use of lasers or endoscopic equipment for complicated surgery. Just attending a two-day workshop and acquiring a certificate does not make a doctor sufficiently expert in using this technology, and a number of mishaps have been reported that have been due to operator inexperience.
- **Use of technology as defensive medicine,** i.e., to protect the doctor from being sued, rather than using it because it is needed for the patient's welfare.

Thus the crucial question arises: What can you do to protect yourself from being a victim of medical technology misuse? The answer is: make sure you are well informed, so that you can judge the technology and its relevance to you for yourself. For example, the National Institutes of Health (NIH) produces consensus statements in which leading medical experts from all over the world are invited to discuss the pros and cons of all the technological options available for dealing with a particular medical problem, essentially in order to guide doctors as to the appropriateness of the latest technologies. Using the information gleaned from such statements or obtained from other sources intelligently, in cooperation with your doctor, will ensure that medical technology is utilized appropriately to provide the best possible care for your problem.

doctor who lives in the rural area, may not be as tuned in to new treatments or even have the latest equipment as a doctors at a major, urban hospital. A second opinion can also serve as a quality check—to make sure you're really getting the most current and most effective treatment. There is no straight-forward answer for when you need a second opinion. You should evaluate your situation to determine what is best for *you*.

There are a number of important questions that you should always ask your physician so that you can make the best choice. The following questions can help you build up a reservoir of medical information to assist you in your decision-making process regarding a particular treatment:

- How much will this treatment improve my chances of getting well? (In other words, what are the benefits?)

- How much risk is involved in this treatment, and what kind of risk is it?
- How long will the treatment take?
- How much will this treatment cost?
- Does undertaking this treatment eliminate other options?
- Are there other options if this treatment fails?

Talk to your physician when you are deciding on what treatment you wish to follow. You should always identify certain vital factors about your treatment before beginning. Unfortunately, not all relationships work out. If worse comes to worse, be prepared to begin the hunt for another primary care physician. For example:
- Time requirements
- Typical physical stress or discomfort expected
- Emotional pressures exerted
- Risks involved
- Expenditure required

Ultimately, the final decision is yours. You will have to ascertain how much money you can spread; how much physical and emotional stress you can bear; and how much risk you are capable of undertaking, only you know the answer to these topic, and it would be best to talk to your doctor openly about these concerns before continuing with a treatment. The main factors which can influence your decision are as follows:

Medical factors:
- Diagnosis (or lack of one)
- Quality and availability of medical care
- Success rate of the treatment
- Level of technology required

Personal factors:
- Age
- Time commitment needed for treatment
- Feelings, both physical and emotional
- Job and career priorities
- Financial resources
- Ethical and religious concerns

- Family and friends' reactions
- Other obligations and commitments
- Willingness to change lifestyle
- Aggressive or low-key approach to resolution

After carefully taking the above factors into consideration and consulting with the doctor you trust, there should be no surprises, and you should be confident in the treatment you choose because your doctor clearly stated all the advantages, as well as disadvantages and the potential outcomes for every type of treatment. If you follow all these guidelines and are unhappy with an outcome, there will be no one to blame but yourself, because every detail should have been explained by your doctor and he was your own choice!

Research Your Options

There are tools available to help you make your own decisions. You should be happy with your decisions and be comfortable that you have made the best decision for yourself, and completed all the research needed to make this decision. A program that can help you in this process is, for example, the Foundation for Informed Medical Decision Making (www.fimdm.org). FIMDM has developed "shared decision-making programs" for common medical problems (such as breast cancer and hormone replacement therapy) that enable you to make up your own mind while sharing all the pros and cons of various treatments.

Do not forget to visit the library—after all, librarians are professional information specialists. Next to an extensive and leisurely consultation with your doctor, or a friend who is a doctor, the library and the Internet are the best places to get your questions answered. An online library that can answer a lot of your medical questions can be found at www.healthlibrary.com. Also explore other websites, such as www.webmd.com.

If you are unfamiliar with a particular topic, a medical encyclopedia is probably the best choice for gathering information. For an excellent overview of just about any medical condition, ideal guides include *The American Medical Association Encyclopedia of Medicine* and the *British Medical Association Family Guide*. A reliable medical dictionary, such as the *Mosby Medical Encyclopedia* or *Merriam-Webster's Medical Desk Dictionary*, can help you make sense of seemingly convoluted terminology. Another publication, *The Merck Manual* (home edition), is a superb compendium of almost every known disorder and describes causes, symptoms, laboratory test, diagnosis, treatment and prognosis.

Your local library may also be able to provide you with useful medical directories that can guide you to further sources of information. For instance, *The Self-Help Source Book,* which lists more than 700 organizations, can help you find a suitable support group. Also, *The Consumer Health Information Source Book* provides information on clearing houses, useful books, and other resources, while the three-volume *Medical and Health Information Directory* lists various organizations, publications, libraries and health services.

If you possess a computer, you can use CD-ROMs effectively to research your problem. Two worthwhile CD-ROMs are the *American Medical Association Family Medical Guide* and the *Mayo Clinic Family Health Encyclopedia*. One advantage of CDs over books is that they offer you computer graphics and even video clips.

If you are looking for information on a specific topic, you need to use one of the Internet's search engines, such as Google (www.google.com). Simply type in the terms ("keywords") you are looking for, and the engine will point you to the relevant information. (A warning for novices: You may also be inundated by a flood of garbage, so you will need to carefully sift through what you find.) There are many useful sites which provide consumer health information. For example, www.healthanswers.com has a superb collection of patient information leaflets on thousands of topics. The remarkable feature about locating a useful site is that it will often have a wide range of links, which will, in turn, point you to other helpful documents, from which you can retrieve even more information.

The Internet offers a number of additional options for acquiring more information on specific topics. There are electronic mailing lists available on many diseases (for example, cancer-l deals with cancer). You can sign up for this by visiting www.pslgroup.com/dg/3d722.htm) that allow you to network with people from all over the world, so that you can keep yourself updated. You can also send out emails to leading medical clinics and medical specialists from all over the world, many of whom will be happy to reply to you—free! There are also special-interest Usenet news groups (for example, www.sci.med.aids.org deals with AIDS), so that you can "talk" to thousands of people from all over the globe who may be facing similar problems!

No matter what your final decision on your treatment is, be sure you are confident that it is the best course of treatment for you!

PART II

SELECTING A HEALTHCARE PLAN

CHAPTER 4

WHAT ARE YOUR OPTIONS?

S ELECTING THE RIGHT HEALTH PLAN should be taken very seriously. It can seem overwhelming to most individuals to choose the right insurance company, especially if you do not have an employer-sponsored health insurance. Simply follow this one rule: until it is broken down part by part, do not purchase it!

In this chapter you will find tips that will help you find the plan that is best for you as well as tips on how to compare the different types of plans you may be confronted with during your search.

How to Begin Your Search

You should know specifically what you want and need, since there are a myriad of health plans offer that offer different benefits. This will require some investigation of the insurance plan as well as your personal needs. The key to choosing a plan is knowing which one will both fit into your budget and best fit you and your family's health needs. For example, perhaps you need a plan that offers comprehensive coverage for young children. Or maybe you need a plan that addresses the chronic health conditions of a family member.

If your health coverage is provided by your employer, you can seek advice from a professional in your employee benefits office, which may be your company's human resources department or the company representative for your company's health plan. Be sure to find out when the next open enrollment is scheduled, at which time you can switch plans. Also, you can call the insurance companies to ask questions. Two key issues to consider when choosing between plans are cost and choice. For example, a fee-for-service plan will typically give you more freedom to choose physicians (including specialists), hospitals, and other healthcare providers than will managed care plans. The flip side is that the cost of care may be at a premium. On the other hand, managed care plans, which include PPOs, HMOs, and POS plans, work with doctors, hospitals, and other healthcare providers that they—not patients—have chosen in order to offer services at a lower cost.

When considering a new health plan, ask the following basic questions:
- Which hospitals are covered by the plan?
- Are there network and out-of-network provisions in the plan?
- What are the standard copayments?
- What is the deductible?
- Is there an out-of-pocket maximum?
- Do I need a referral from a primary care provider to see a specialist, or can I self-refer?
- Is there an annual or lifetime limit on coverage?

You'll also want to find out what specific benefits are offered by the new plan. Ask about coverage for:
- Physical exams and health screenings
- Preventive care, such as flu shots and mammograms
- Specialists
- Hospitalization and emergency care
- Laboratory and diagnostic costs
- Prescription drugs
- Eye exams and vision care
- Dental care, including orthodontia

You also may wish to ask about:
- Mental health counseling and care
- Drug and alcohol abuse services
- Smoking cessation
- Care for chronic illnesses and related medical supplies
- Physical and occupational therapy
- Home healthcare

• Alternative or complementary healthcare
• Experimental treatments (clinical trials)

You might also want to ask about specialty care. This is in case you suddenly come down with a serious disease or illness, which most people do not take into consideration unless they have a family history of a particular disease (which is very important to consider), but, if it were to occur (that is, you or someone in your family coming down with a serious illness that you could not predict), you would want to seek the best medical care. For example, patients travel to the Cleveland Clinic from across the United States and from more than a hundred countries around the world to seek specialty care.

When you are choosing among health plans, ask what type of coverage is available for specialty care. In addition, be sure to find out if specialty care from an out-of-state medical center is covered.

Another consideration is convenience. Find out how far you will have to travel for care. Ask about the availability of your primary care physician. For example, are you able to be seen in a reasonable time, or must you wait months for an appointment? Ask how the plan addresses medical care (including vision and dental) if you are far from home.

The quality of care is an important consideration, and asking the right questions will help you determine which hospitals and physicians you prefer. See the section "How to Choose a Doctor" on page 3 for details.

Keep in mind that anything is possible, so the same way that you negotiate for a car or a house or with your doctor, you can negotiate with your insurance company. If the company is unwilling to negotiate, it is not the company for you. There are plenty out there, so look for a new one.

Finding a Plan in Your Area

You should begin your search by discovering what is available in your state. An organization that can be helpful in this process is the National Association of Insurance Commissioners (NAIC). This association helps regulate the insurance industry and protects consumers by ensuring that insurance companies and health plans act in accordance with the insurance laws. They can assist you in the decision-making process or can even refer you to an impartial broker (discussed later in this chapter).

Simply because of your state of residency, you may have a low price available to you. Some states have guaranteed-issue laws, which forbid insurance companies from rejecting people based on the condition of their health. Other states have a "community rating" system, which requires insurers to charge everyone the same rates, regardless of health. This system also sometimes limits the insurance company's ability to raise premiums, which sometimes has the unfortunately side effect that those who are healthy pay more in health insurance than they would if they lived in another state.

New Jersey is an example of a "community rating" system. Everyone pays the same rate for similar coverage, whether he is a 27-year-old triathlete or a 55-year-old who has had quadruple-bypass surgery. The benefit of this system is that everyone is able to buy insurance; the downside is that it is more expensive than in Pennsylvania, where individuals are able to buy comparable health insurance coverage for a little less.

On the other hand, California is a state with a highly competitive health insurance market and no community-rating or guaranteed-issue laws. This benefits individuals who are in good health, because the competitive market drives prices down.

There is, unfortunately, no sure route to finding affordable health coverage on your own because of how variable plans are from state to state. For example, if you happen to live in a rural area, you'll have very few choices of health insurance plans. You won't always be able to save money with an HMO if there aren't enough people in your area to make it economical. Association plans, which sometimes offer good deals, are not available in several states. Also, your state may limit your options for raising deductibles or cutting back on coverage to lower the price tag.

Finding a plan that works to your advantage on your own can be long and tedious, which is why some people may opt to have someone do the research for them. This person is called an insurance broker or salesman.

About Brokers

A broker is someone who can help explain what you are getting from your insurance as well as make sure that you and the members of your family are in the correct plan. Brokers not only will help you shop for price, they'll also know if a company has a reputation for raising premiums or hassling policyholders who file claims. If necessary, a broker can find a group for you to join or help you sign up for your state's high-risk pool.

If your potential insurance broker makes it seem complicated and too difficult to understand, run for the hills. Usually, there is a reason that he is being unclear: he has something to hide. Your insurance information should be crystal clear and very simple to understand. After all, your healthcare premium is usually the second or third largest monthly payment you will be making, next to your home and car, so choose wisely.

Do not let an insurance agent or broker tell you what you need; instead, make the broker match your needs. Read the fine print in every plan you are considering, and ask questions. Just because the broker tells you that liver transplantation is covered does not make him responsible if the statement turns out to not be true. Remember to document (in writing) everything you discuss with the broker, especially luxury items such as dental care, eye care, and organ transplantation.

> *I developed hepatitis C through a blood transfusion at birth. Subsequently, I developed liver cirrhosis years later, only to find out that my HMO plan did not cover liver transplantation in the event of liver failure from hepatitis C. I was then denied coverage by three alternative health plans due to this preexisting condition. I had to raise the money independently, negotiating a flat fee of $90,000 with the transplant center and hospital. I am still in litigation, trying to recover expenses over the denials and lack of coverage, but I am not sure if I will be able to recover any of it.*
>
> *—Helen Peabody, age 28*

Finding a broker can be difficult, but once you find one you are comfortable with, you won't have to worry about keeping up with your ever-changing healthcare policy. Many life and auto insurance agents don't deal in health insurance because the rules are complicated and the commissions are low. However, they may be able to refer you to a specialist.

The National Association of Health Underwriters, www.nahu.org, or your local state insurance commissioner may be able to put you in touch with a reputable broker in your area. The key is getting a broker that has a "large book," whom you trust, and who is experienced enough to know what policies are best for your individual needs. The right broker can save you a lot of time and headaches in the future.

Comparing Plans

In the following chapters, you'll find in-depth explanations of each of the different plans available on the market. Some won't fit your needs or will not be available for you to purchase. To make this process a bit easier for you and to narrow down which plans may work for your needs, here is a brief introduction to each type of insurance plan.

HMOs, or health maintenance organizations, tend to be a good deal if you are in a good market, are relatively healthy, and want the one-stop-shopping structure of a staff/group. This plan tends to have fewer bells and whistles than most insurance plans and covers the more general medical

What Plans Are Options for Me?		
Age	**Criteria**	**Plans Available**
Younger than 20	No insurance coverage by family	SCHIPs (State Children's Health Insurance Plan) Medicaid Medicare
	(else)	Private Insurance*
20-64	Fatal kidney problems or Disability for more than 24 months	Medicare
	Low income as determined by the state	Medicaid
	(else)	Private Insurance*
65+	Low income as determined by the state	Medicaid Medicare
	(else)	Medicare Private Insurance*
*Private Insurance includes all privately funded plans, such as HMOs, PPOs, HRAs, and HSAs.		

concerns; everything is in black and white and straightforward. This is why the HMO less complicated to understand. for more information about HMOs, see Chapter 6.

PPOs (preferred provider organizations) are associations of doctors who have contracted with an insurance company to provide services at a discounted fee; thus there is a little gray area when dealing with the insurance companies. Because of the flexibility of choosing your doctor as well as specialists in the network, there tend to be fewer delays in getting the care that is needed, as well as fewer difficulties getting the most appropriate care. There also tend to be fewer cases of being forced to change doctors. However, due to this flexibility, there may be a greater number of problems in billing and in understanding their benefits. For more information about PPOs, see Chapter 7.

POS (point of service) is offered within some HMO plans. Basically, this offers you greater flexibility in choosing healthcare providers by allowing you to use doctors that are not within the HMO network. If your doctor makes a referral outside the network, the plan will pay all or most of the bill. If you refer yourself to a provider outside the network and the service is covered by the plan, you will have to pay coinsurance. For more information about POS plans, see Chapter 7.

FFS (fee-for-service) plans offer a scope of services provided where you are generally free to seek your provider. Not all services may be covered and there is a maximum reimbursement specified for most services if not all. This plan is generally less expensive than a PPO and has more options than an HMO. For more information about FFS plans, see Chapter 7.

Medicare is a federal health insurance program offered to all Americans age 65 or older and people with certain disabilities. In many parts of the country, people covered by Medicare now have a choice between managed care and indemnity plans. They can also switch their plan for any reason. However, they must notify the plan or the local Social Security office, and the change may not take effect for up to 30 days. Call your local Social Security office or your state office on aging to find out what is available in your area. For more information about Medicare, see Chapter 8.

Medicaid is a good option if you are considered "low-income" by your state (especially children and pregnant women), and disabled people. Medicaid is a joint federal-state health insurance program that is run by the states. In some cases, states require people covered under Medicaid to join managed care plans. Insurance plans and state regulations differ, so check with your state Medicaid office to learn more. For more information about Medicaid, see Chapter 9.

One of the more popular military health plans is TRICARE. TRI-CARE is a regionally managed healthcare program for active-duty, activated National Guard and reserves, retired members of the uniformed services, their families, and survivors. TRICARE brings together the healthcare resources of the Army, Navy, and Air Force and supplements them with networks of civilian healthcare professionals to provide better access and high-quality service while maintaining the capability to support military operations.

Active-duty, National Guard, and reserve service members are automatically enrolled in TRICARE Prime. However military dependents and retirees must choose from a variety of TRICARE options one that best suits their needs. For more information on coverage in the military, see Chapter 10.

FSAs/HSAs/HRAs (Flexible Spending Accounts/Health Savings Accounts/Health Reimbursement Accounts) are a pretty good option for small businesses. They are not health insurance plans but special tax-sheltered savings accounts you can use to accumulate funds for medical bills. The rules for these plans are complicated, and each plan is slightly different, so study them carefully. For more information about FSAs/HSAs/HRAs, see Chapter 11.

COBRA coverage tends to be a good deal if you're in poor health or in a market with few choices or you want to stick with your current doctors. But because group plans often have more bells and whistles than you'd buy yourself, you might find a better deal by shopping on your own. For more information about COBRA, see Chapter 12.

Research Your Options

No matter which plan you choose, you will examine a benefits summary or an outline of coverage. This may include a description of policy benefits, exclusions, and provisions that makes it easier to understand a particular policy and compare it with others.

Take the time to evaluate each plan's coverage and features, taking into account exclusions, limitations, and the freedom to choose healthcare providers. Find out how much you'll end up paying out of pocket in the form of copayments, coinsurance, and deductibles, because even relatively

---

When to Join Your Spouse's Healthcare Plan

Many married couples maintain separate health insurance coverage even though it may not be cost-effective to do so. Examine both your own coverage and your spouse's to see if it makes sense for either of you to join the other's plan. Keep in mind that most plans allow you to add a spouse to your plan within a certain time period after you get married (e.g., 30 days). Otherwise, you may have to wait for the plans' annual open enrollment period.

---

small amounts of money can really add up if you make frequent visits to your doctor. There is a lot of room for negotiating with insurance companies, especially on an annual basis when insurance companies launch new products.

Most good insurance companies allow plenty of room for negotiating because they understand that the healthcare industry is constantly changing—and so are your needs. This is why it is important to find out if there is an appeal process before signing on. Being able to appeal will give you the opportunity to explain to the insurance company why you need a certain procedure or treatment that is not covered by the insurance. Most appeal decisions can have you waiting more than 30 days. If waiting this amount of time would pose a serious threat to your health, such as loss of life, limb, or major bodily function, ask for an "expedited" appeal and explain why you need a quick decision. The general rule is that the plan must respond within five days unless it is specified differently in your plan.

In addition to an appeals process, be sure your insurance policy covers what you need and may need in the future. Do you want coverage for your whole family or just yourself? Are you concerned with preventive care and checkups? Or would you be comfortable in a managed care setting, which might restrict your choice somewhat but give you broad coverage and convenience? When you are searching for a plan, try these simple steps:

- **Check out prices on the Web. In order to get started on some initial quotes, websites such as** eHealthInsurance (www.ehealthinsurance.com) may be able to help, although the information in some states is limited and some companies may be excluded. Some other insurance companies, such as BlueCross/

BlueShield, may have all of their plans and benefits listed on their website, making it easier to compare. Another site, Digital Insurance (www.digitalinsurance. com), lists prices for different groups of health insurance companies. These sites are most useful in competitive markets such as California but won't help much in Maine and other restrictive states. Taking a peek at the sites and knowing what else is available may be worth your while even if you're happy with your current plan. You can find several options online through www.ehealthinsurance.com. Be sure you understand that not every insurance company has a website, and just because a company has a website, it doesn't mean it is the best for you. Use the information you find on the Internet as preliminary research material; then call the company and ask it to elaborate on what you have found on its website. I would also recommend locating your state insurance commissioner in the department of insurance for more information and another opinion on the Web by going to www.naic. org.state_web_map.htm or by calling 202-624-7790 and asking for the number of your state's commissioner. You never know what new plans are coming out in your area as well as new rules that may change the benefits of your current plan.

- **Visit your state insurance department's website.** You may find a list of companies selling individual coverage in your state, including those that aren't handled by brokers. For example, many BlueCross/BlueShield plans—often one of the few choices available in highly restrictive states—prefer to deal directly with customers or offer such low commissions that they aren't worth a broker's time. The insurance department may provide shopping tips for your state, as well as insurance company complaint records. The website that can direct you to your state insurance department is www.nahu.org.

- **Look into your state's insurance pool** if you have been turned down for coverage because of your health problems. In Texas, for example, anyone who can't get coverage elsewhere must be covered by the high-risk pool, although prices can be steep. States with guaranteed coverage, such as New Jersey, don't have high-risk pools because regular health insurance companies are required to cover everyone.

- **Consider taking advantage of federal COBRA legislation.** If you left a company that provided group coverage and your previous employer has 20 or more employees, the company is required by law to let you continue your group coverage for up to 18 months. Some states have similar laws for smaller employers. You generally foot the entire bill yourself, plus up to 2 percent in administrative charges, which can increase your costs considerably.
- **Form your own small group.** Even rates for tiny groups are more competitive and offer lower prices than do individual policies. For example, in New Jersey you can form a group with as few as two employees, including yourself, as long as each employee works a minimum of 25 hours per week and you pay the employer's share of Social Security taxes for your workers. Group policies can cost 20 to 50 percent less than individual coverage. In Washington, another state with few choices in individual health insurance, self-employed people can form a group of one and have a much wider selection with more competitive prices. But you have to submit tax forms that prove you really are a business.
- **Join an association that has group coverage.** In some areas, such as Rochester, New York, the local chamber of commerce offers some health insurance options worth investigating. You can find your local chamber of commerce's information online at www.2chambers.com.

If you're on your own and in good health, you'll have the toughest time finding affordable coverage in New Jersey, New York, and Vermont. In these states, the law requires that insurers have to charge everyone the same premiums. Such a combination adds up to little competition and high prices.

States where affordable insurance is easier to come by because there is no community rating include: Alabama, Alaska, Arizona, Arkansas, California, Colorado, Connecticut, Delaware, Florida, Georgia, Illinois, Kansas, Maryland, Mississippi, Missouri, Montana, Nebraska, Nevada, North Carolina, Oklahoma, South Carolina, Tennessee, and Texas.

Here is a partial list of coverage to consider when comparing health insurance plans:

- Inpatient hospital services
- Outpatient surgery

- Physician visits (in the hospital)
- Office visits
- Skilled nursing care
- Prescription drugs
- Medical tests and x-rays
- Mental healthcare
- Drug and alcohol abuse treatment
- Home healthcare visits
- Rehabilitation facility care
- Physical therapy
- Speech therapy
- Maternity care
- Hospice care
- Chiropractic treatment
- Preventive care and checkups
- Well-baby care
- Dental care
- Other covered services

Ask these questions when reviewing potential plans:
- How much is the premium? When will I have to pay it (every month, quarter, or year)?
- Are there any medical service limits, exclusions, or preexisting conditions that will affect you or your family?
- What types of utilization review, pre authorization, or certification procedures are included?
- Are there any discounts available for good health or healthy behaviors (e.g., not smoking)?
- How much is the annual deductible (per person and per family)?
- What coinsurance or copayments apply?
- What percentage payment is expected after the deductible is met?
- What is the copay or percentage of coinsurance per office visit?
- What is the copay or percentage of coinsurance for "wellness" care (including well-baby care, annual eye exam, physical, etc.)?
- What is the percentage of copay or coinsurance for inpatient hospital care?

Preexisting Conditions and HIPAA

Many people worry about their health coverage when they have preexisting conditions, especially when they change jobs. However, the Health Insurance Portability and Accountability Act of 1996 (HIPAA) (see www.hipaa.org) helps ensure continued health insurance coverage for employees and their dependents despite preexisting medical conditions. It also helps to reduce healthcare fraud and abuse, enforce standards for health information, and guarantee the security and privacy of your health information. The bottom line is that HIPAA offers you protection.

In most cases, an insurer will impose only one 12-month waiting period for any preexisting condition treated or diagnosed in the previous six months. Your prior health insurance coverage will be credited toward the preexisting condition exclusion period as long as you have maintained continuous coverage without a break of more than 62 days. Pregnancy is not considered a preexisting condition, and newborns and adopted children who are covered within 30 days are not subject to the 12-month waiting period.

However, do not let your coverage lapse for more than 62 days. If you do go beyond the 62-day period, chances are your insurance premiums will increase, even if you were under a "temporary" insurance plan at that time. Keep in mind that most "temporary" health insurance plans do not qualify as standard health insurance, so a lapse in coverage will count against you when you sign up for a permanent insurance. This does not apply if you were covered under an insurance policy such as COBRA (see page 139 for more information on this).

Waiting periods can be a bit frustrating, but as long as you have the information on what is legally allowed, you will be able to make sure your rights are being respected. For example, if you have had group health coverage for two years and you switch jobs and go to another plan, that new health plan cannot impose a preexisting condition exclusion period. This means that the insurance company cannot deny claims pertaining to an existing condition at the time you enroll or purchase your health insurance. Typically, it will deny all claims pertaining to that condition for a certain period of time. If you have had prior coverage of only eight months, you may be subject to a four-month preexisting condition exclusion period when you switch jobs. If you've never been covered by an employer's group plan and you get a job that offers such coverage, you may be subject to a 12-month preexisting condition waiting period.

Federal laws are also in place to make it easier for you to get individual insurance in certain situations, including if you have left a job where you had group health insurance or had another plan for more than 18 months without a break of more than 62 days. For more information, you can go to the Department of Labor website at www.dol.gov or the Health Insurance Portability and Accountability Act website under Centers for Medicare and Medicaid Services at www.cms.hhs.gov/HIPAAGenInfo/02_TheHIPAA LawandMore.asp#TopOfPage.

If you have not been covered under a group plan and have found it difficult to get insurance on your own because of your preexisting condition, check with your state's insurance department at www.naic.org/state_web_map.htm to see if your state has a risk pool. Similar to risk pools for automobile insurance, these can provide health insurance for people who cannot get it elsewhere.

Another thing to keep in mind that some states, such as Maryland and Washington, have no medical underwriting and do not discriminate based on preexisting conditions. Medical underwriting is the screening of prospective healthcare plan members out of a plan on the basis of health or preexisting medical condition. This has been a battle for many years and will probably always remain one. Unfortunately, I have even witnessed people determining their residency on state underwriting due to a family member's "preexisting condition." So be sure to do some extra due diligence if you or a family member has a preexisting condition; it will save you a lot of money and headaches in the end.

In conclusion, know that there are organizations such as HIPPA that can help define your rights if you get into a bind and are unclear about health insurance rules. Just be sure to do as much research as possible, organize your thoughts, and write all your questions down, even those that you "sort of" understand. When you contact an organization such as HIPPA, be sure to request documentation of the answers or ask the representative where it is located. If you ever need to go back to review the information for your own understanding or explain a health insurance issue to your insurance company, which does not seem as familiar with the federal laws governing health insurance rights, you will have it on hand. Remember, HIPPA is there to protect you.

Get the Most from Your Health Insurance

The easiest and best way to get the most out of your health insurance is to know what and who your insurance policy covers before you need to use it. Your health insurance may cover more than you think. Nowadays, insurance companies often provide benefits designed to help you stay safe and healthy, called "preventive medicine," which will be described later. For example, you may receive discounts on vitamins, alternative medicines, health club memberships, or bike helmets.

You may also be surprised at the range of coverage your health plan offers. for instance, it may cover dental care for young children, chiropractic care, and acupuncture. Read your plan membership materials to find out what products and services are available through your health plan before you pay for them on your own.

If You Are Denied Coverage

There may be a time when you find yourself filing an appeal because you have been denied coverage. When you appeal, be sure you have read and fully understand the terms of the EOC or SPD. Next, consult with your PCP. You may want to consider a second opinion if your insurance will allow it (these guidelines should also be stated in the EOC or SPD).

If the denial is by your health insurance plan, contact the department that made the decision and calmly ask for an explanation in writing. If the reason for the denial is that the care is not "medically necessary," or if another treatment is suggested, you will need to explain why the treatment you seek is the most appropriate one for your condition. Doing so may require you to do some medical research to learn more about your condition and treatment options.

A Center for Health Care Rights can be located in most states and can provide you with the information you may need to appeal. Most are advocates for Medicare beneficiaries but can also be helpful to those who are not enrolled in Medicare. For example, the Center for Health Care Rights in California ". . . is a California-based nonprofit organization dedicated to assuring consumer access to quality healthcare through information, education, counseling, advocacy, and research programs. The Center informs its efforts to represent consumers in public and private policy forums by the direct service it provides to individual consumers." The CHCR can be found online at www.healthcarerights.org. This includes some important links as well as guidance on health insurance concerns, including sample letters for healthcare consumers on common healthcare issues.

It is imperative that you keep up with your "insurance rules" due to the fact that healthcare policy changes so frequently throughout the year. A good rule of the thumb is to double-check your policy and verify what is in your EOC or SPD with a representative before you go in for a procedure to be sure you are covered for the procedure and verify the guidelines, thus freeing yourself of any confusion down the line. Be sure to document whom you spoke with as well as the date.

If you do not use your plan frequently, review it annually with the members of your plan, or with your broker, to be sure the EOC or SPD is still consistent with what you originally signed up for and evaluate your usage. You may find that either your health status has changed or the plan has. If so, you will need to review other plans. Keep in mind that you want a health plan that accommodates your health rather than one that forces you to accommodate your health to your plan.

Conclusion

If you have healthcare coverage at work or through a trade or professional association or a union, you are almost certainly enrolled under a group contract. Generally, the contract is between the group and the insurer, and your employer has done some comparison shopping before offering the plan to the employees. Nevertheless, while some employers offer only one plan, some offer more than one. Compare your potential plans carefully!

If you are buying individual insurance or any form of insurance that you purchase directly, read and compare the policies you are considering before you buy one, and make sure you understand all of the provisions. Marketing or sales literature is no substitute for the actual policy. Read the policy itself before you buy.

- **Ask for a summary** of each policy's benefits or an outline of coverage. Good agents and good insurance companies want you to know what you are buying. Don't be afraid to ask your benefits manager or insurance agent to explain anything that is unclear.
- **Ask for the insurance company's rating.** There are several websites that grade insurance companies in your area. The National Committee for Quality Assurance, whose focus is to "measure the

quality of America's Healthcare" offers an array of information of the satisfaction of healthcare policies in your area on http://hprc.ncqa.org/frameset.asp. You may also call the agency at 202-955-3500. The A. M. Best Company at www.ambest.com and Standard & Poor's Corporation at http://info.insure.com/ratings/profiles/ also provide health insurance ratings that can help in your decision making process.

- **You may have 30 days to return the policy** and get your money back if it does not meet your needs. This is called a "free look." According to some healthcare plans, your doctor may have to receive permission from the provider in order to make a referral. This can potentially delay a healthcare problem that needs immediate attention. If you believe this is the case, contact your doctor or your health plan's or medical group's customer service department for assistance right away.

- **Notify your health insurance company as soon as possible if there is a serious situation.** If you receive emergency care or if you are admitted to a hospital for emergency services, whether it is within or outside the plan's network, the standard for notification is 24 to 48 hours. Some plans will require you to notify your primary care physician. Others may be satisfied with a call to a customer service representative with an explanation of the care needed, where you received it, and what treatments or services were provided. In most cases, you will need follow-up care. A health plan representative will probably arrange for follow-up care in another facility or at your home if the hospital where you received emergency care does not participate in your health plan. All plans must cover emergency care, but it is necessary to follow your plan's guidelines in order to avoid problems in the future.

As you can see from the above, every plan has a different set of rules, and it is up to you to read through them and understand them. If you do not understand the benefits, be sure to call the insurance company and have it clarify them; don't let it brush you off by saying "Look in the benefits package we sent you." If you feel the answer provided was incomplete, ask to speak to a supervisor; be sure to document the names and contact information of every person you speak with just in case you need to reference them later on. Never wait until something happens to start your investigation, and always double-check with the insurance company for new packages every so often, especially when it is time to renew. This can save you a lot of time, money, and annoyance in the long run.

CHAPTER 5

THE LINGO OF HEALTHCARE PLANS

MOST OF US WILL AGREE that trying to understand health insurance feels as if it requires a college degree. In most cases, even the doctors providing the healthcare find the terms and conditions of the insurance plans difficult to understand, let alone an insurance broker who does not have a medical degree. You can usually ask your doctor to translate a diagnosis into terms you can understand, but it's much harder to get an insurance broker to do the same. Understanding the lingo of your healthcare coverage is crucial and even time-sensitive, because you often will not have a second chance to reconsider after open season (the time period when you are allowed to change your policy without penalties). Reading the fine print of your healthcare plan can and potentially will save you bundles of cash.

A health plan agreement, contract, or summary should be given to you as soon as you join the health plan, and you definitely should have been given time enough to review the document in detail. This is usually called "Evidence of Coverage" (EOC) or "Summary Plan Description" (SPD). It explains your healthcare benefits, your coverage limits, the health plan's policies and procedures, and what costs you will have to pay.

As soon as you have the EOC or SPD in hand, you'll be able to see the details of your potential health plan's coverage. Typically, they will also include a list of definitions to make it easier to read. If there are any terms you do not understand, be sure to mark them and ask your health plan customer service representative to explain them to you. Many healthcare plans define terms differently, so it is important to fully understand the provider's definition. We have a short glossary of the more popular and potentially cost saving terms in Appendix C.

Beware of the Deductible

The deductible is the amount of money in addition to your monthly insurance monthly premium that you pay before the insurance company starts paying for your medical expenses. This can be a bit confusing until you realize that the deductible is cumulative.

For example, your first doctor appointment of the year is in March. Your deductable under your health plan is $250. The bill for your general practitioner totals $180. You are responsible for the full amount of the bill at this point because your total medical expenses have not yet reached $250. You return for a follow-up visit, resulting in a $120 bill. Because you have already spent $180 toward your owed deductible, you only owe $70 of the $120 ($70 + $180 = $250). If your deductible had been $500, you would continue to be responsible for all your medical bills until you reach the $500 mark. Obviously, if you are a healthy individual who rarely visits the doctor, it is to your advantage to obtain an insurance policy with a lower deductible for outpatient visits and a higher deductible for hospital and catastrophic coverage.

When you are paying for your bill, remember that the deductible is paid to your insurance company and not to your doctor. If you are an individual who visits the doctor frequently, it's likely you will have a high deductible. On January 1, this process restarts. Do not assume that your insurance company is paying your physician a percentage of your deductible toward your bill. At times mistakes are made in the initial diagnosis or in the coding, there may be changes in the policy that you may be unaware of, and so on The bill collectors do not know the "history" of the billing problem; they just see an overdue bill, which may lead to late payment fees and additional charges.

It is always better to pay your bill in full and deal with reimbursement from your insurance company later. Remember to always obtain an itemized copy of your bill at the time of service and consult with the office manager or billing manager regarding how much of the total will be your responsibility. This will help eliminate any confusion when the reimbursement comes from the insurance company at a later date because you will have a copy of the bill and have a better idea of what was actually reimbursed if the billing manager explains it to you and be able to make arrangements with the billing manager if there are any discrepancies without being penalized by the insurance company.

Sometimes you can get so caught up in choosing an insurance policy based on the monthly premium that you overlook the deductible. Actually, you should look at both together. For example, an insurance premium of $20 more per month with a $250 deductible will be far less costly overall than a slightly cheaper premium with a $500 deductible.

Pharmaceutical Deductible

When you head to the pharmacy to fill a prescription, the deductible you pay has nothing to do with the cumulative outpatient or inpatient care deductible. Don't make the mistake of overlooking the additional coverage needed for your medications when selecting an insurer. Also, do not attempt to hide medication information when you are applying for insurance. Insurance companies incorporate all factors of medical history, medication history and use and have access to *all* your information. They will find out.

Deductibles for pharmaceutical coverage work similarly to that of regular medical coverage. After paying the deductible amount (usually around $100 per year), the insured is responsible only for the copay amount for each prescription (usually $10 to $30 per prescription). However, if you suffer from a chronic illness and spend thousands of dollars per year on medication, it's to your advantage to seek a higher deductible, as obtaining a lower deductible (i.e., $100), will result in the insurance company compensating with a much higher overall monthly premium. In other words, you will probably be paying more per month even if your deductible is lower.

For example, you may pay a $100-per-month premium with a deductible of $2,500 per year (which means you are responsible for the first $2,500 of your medical expenses, even if the insurance company covers them) as opposed to paying a $224-per-month premium with a $1,000-per-year deductible. A rule of thumb: Never request a drug plan with a low deductible ($250/year or less) if your insured retail drug costs exceed $2,000 per year. To maintain more manageable premiums, only healthy individuals with low medication requirements should request a deductible of less than $250 per year, since their medication costs will rarely exceed this amount over the course of a year. If this is overlooked and you are issued a higher deductible (over $500 per year), you will end up paying out of pocket for all your medications, usually around $250 or less per year, which is definitely not to your advantage.

An additional option for obtaining cheaper medications is through wholesalers such as Costco, Sam's Club or Wal-Mart. Sometimes copay amounts at retail pharmacies may exceed the actual wholesale cost of the drug, especially drugs after the patent has expired (for example, the antiacid medication, Prilosec (Omeprazole) was $3.50 per 20-milligram capsule by prescription and now is $0.68 per 20-milligram capsule, since the patent expired in 2003). I recently filled a prescription for 30 tablets of the antinausea medication Compazine (off patent since 1990) for $12 cash at Costco, whereas using my prescription card at CVS would have cost the $20 copay. So remember to call around and use the Internet as a good resource when finding out the actual cost of a medication. Unfortunately, the lower costs do not apply to newer drugs; however, some of the older medications are often just as affective and a fraction of the cost.

Common Terms Used for Independent Health Insurance Policies

While basic health insurance provides benefits when you have a covered condition that requires hospitalization, there are other policies available that may supplement your insurance.

Your basic benefits typically include room and board and other hospital services, surgery, physicians' nonsurgical services performed in a hospital, expenses for diagnostic x-rays and laboratory tests, and room and board in an extended care facility. Benefits for hospital room and board may be a per day dollar amount or all or part of the hospital's daily rate for a semiprivate room. Benefits for surgery typically are listed, showing the maximum benefit for each type of surgical procedure.

- **Hospital-surgical policies** provide "first-dollar" coverage. That means that there is no deductible, or amount that you have to pay, for a covered medical expense. Most other policies include a small deductible. Keep in mind that hospital-surgical policies usually do not cover lengthy hospitalizations and costly medical care. In the event that you need these types of services, you may incur large expenses that are difficult to meet unless you have other insurance.

- **Catastrophic coverage** pays hospital and medical expenses above a certain deductible. This can provide additional protection if you hold either a hospital-surgical policy or a major medical policy with a lower-than-adequate lifetime limit. These policies typically contain a very high deductible ($15,000 or more) and a maximum lifetime limit high enough to cover the costs of catastrophic illness.
- **Specified policies** provide benefits only if you get the specific disease or group of diseases named in the policy. For example, a policy might cover only medical care for cancer. Because benefits are limited in amount, these policies are not a substitute for broad medical coverage. Nor are specified disease policies available in every state. The following website can help get you started on finding an insurance company that will cover the management of your specific condition: www.ncqa.org/programs/accreditation/DM/dmaccredstatus.htm. In addition, you may elect to contact a specific agency to help locate an insurance plan for your condition. For example, if you have osteoporosis, both the National Institute on Aging at 800-222-2225 or www.nih.gov/nia or the National Osteoporosis Foundation at 202-223-2226 or www.nof.org can help locate an insurance plan that specializes in managing your condition.
- **Hospital indemnity insurance or a medical gap plan** pays you a specified amount of cash benefits for each day that you are hospitalized, generally up to a designated number of days. These cash benefits are paid directly to you, can be used for any purpose, and may be useful in meeting out-of-pocket expenses not covered by other insurance.

Hospital indemnity policies are frequently available directly from insurance companies by mail as well as through insurance agents. You will find that these policies offer many choices, so be sure to ask questions and find the right plan to meet your needs.

Some policies contain limitations on preexisting medical conditions that you may have before your insurance takes effect. Others contain an elimination period, which means that benefits will not be paid until after you have been hospitalized for a specified number of days. When you apply for the policy, you may be allowed to choose among two or three elimination periods, with different premiums for each. Although you can reduce your premiums by choosing a longer elimination period, you should bear in mind that most patients are hospitalized for relatively brief periods of time.

If you purchase a hospital indemnity policy, periodically review it to see if you need to increase your daily benefits to keep pace with rising health-care costs.

- **Disability insurance** provides you with income if illness or injury prevents you from being able to work for an extended period of time. It is an important but often overlooked form of insurance. Please remember that besides for this insurance, there are other possible sources of income if you are disabled. Social Security provides some protection, but only to those who are severely disabled and unable to work at all; workers' compensation provides benefits if the illness or injury is work-related; civil service disability covers federal or state government workers; and automobile insurance may pay benefits if the disability results from an automobile accident. But these sources are limited. To find out if you qualify and possible benefits, go to www.ssa.gov/pubs/10029.html or call 800-772-1213.

- **Short- and long-term disability coverage** are options similar to disability insurance, useful if you are self-employed. You can buy individual disability income insurance policies. Generally, monthly benefits are usually 60 percent of your income at the time of purchase, although cost-of-living adjustments may be available. If you pay premiums for an individual disability policy, the payments you receive under the policy are not subject to income tax. If your employer has paid some or all of the premiums under a group disability policy, some or all of the benefits may be taxable.

Whether you are an employer shopping for a group disability policy or someone thinking of purchasing disability income insurance, you will need to evaluate several different policies.

Some policies pay benefits only if someone is unable to perform the duties of his or her customary occupation, while others pay only if the person can engage in no gainful employment at all. Make sure that you know the insurer's definition of disability. Some policies pay only for accidents, but it's important to be insured for illness, too. Be sure, as you evaluate policies, that both accident and illness are covered.

Benefits may begin anywhere from one to six months or more after the onset of disability. A later starting date can keep your premiums down. Remember, if your policy starts to pay (for example) only two months after the disability begins, you may lose a considerable amount of income.

Benefits may be payable for a period ranging anywhere from one year to a lifetime. Since disability benefits replace income, most people do not need benefits beyond their working years. But it's generally wise to insure at least until age 65 since a lengthy disability threatens financial security much more than a short disability does.

Tax Deductions for Medical Expenses

Tax deductions that are available to you need definition frequently. Your medical expenses can easily add up even without health insurance, and one of the best ways to recover from the out-of-pocket expenses is to write them off on your taxes.

An important thing to note is that you must reach a minimum before you can deduct medical expenses. For example, only medical expenses that are greater than 7.5 percent of your adjusted gross income; this includes wages, interest, income from retirement accounts, capital gains, or alimony received. In the U.S. federal tax system, it is defined as income after certain adjustments are made but before standardized and itemized deductions and personal exemptions are made. See http://en.wikipedia.org/wiki/Adjusted_ Gross_Income for more information.

For example, if my annual salary is $50,000 per year, I can deduct out-of-pocket medical expenses only beyond $3,750. So if I have $5,000 of qualified costs, I am left with a deduction of just $1,250. Even that partial deduction can make a difference. If I'm in the 25 percent bracket, a $1,250 deduction can lower my tax bill by $313.

Be sure to keep the receipts in your tax file throughout the year because you could end up with a surprisingly large deduction if you have a medical emergency or a major expense that isn't covered by insurance. Once you pass that threshold, you can write off other nonreimbursed expenses that are usually too small to qualify.

Am I still eligible if I have a flexible spending account at work?
Even if you contribute the maximum to your flexible spending account at work—generally $2,000 to $3,000 per year—you still may have some left-over expenses to write off. If one year, for example, you spend $20,000 for two rounds of in vitro fertilization that aren't covered by your health insurance, and you pay for $3,000 of the cost from your flexible spending account, then you'll still have $17,000 in unreimbursed medical expenses that could qualify for the tax write-off. If you earn $60,000 per year, you can write off any medical expenses beyond $4,500 (7.5 percent of your adjusted gross income). That still leaves you with $12,500 to write off, which will lower your tax bill by $3,125 if you're in the 25 percent bracket.

Are there ways to exceed the minimum amount legally?
There are several ways of computing your taxes to take advantage of this write-off. If you are married, you (or your spouse) may even pool your medical expenses under one tax return and combine the medical expenses of your dependents in order to allow you to have more of your household's medical expenses, which may take you over the threshold of 7.5 percent of your adjusted gross income (AGI). If you and your spouse each claims your own medical expenses, you will usually end up with a lower combined tax credit than if you had claimed them on one return.

If you are married yet filing separately, the lower-earning spouse should claim your family's medical expenses; however, any medical expenses paid out of a joint checking account in which you and your spouse have the same interest are considered to have been paid equally by each of you.

It may also be possible to shift tax deductions between tax years to take advantage of the 7.5 percent limit. For example, you could prepay your orthodontia bill or pay your January 1 medical insurance on December 31. Consider paying medical expenses in the tax year in which you will have a lower AGI, because the lower your AGI, the greater the allowable medical tax deductions on your tax return. You could also postpone or accelerate elective treatments, and increase the percentage for a particular tax year.

Can I claim the expenses of family members or dependents?
You can claim the medical expenses for family members who were dependent on you for support for that entire tax year and are a resident of the United States, Canada, or Mexico for some part of the tax year. This could include

grandchildren, parents, grandparents, siblings, uncles, aunts, nieces, or nephews. A person generally qualifies as your dependent for purposes of the medical expense deduction if all three of the following requirements are met:

- The person lived in your home for the entire year (365 days) or meets certain relationship requirements as described in IRS Publication 501 or on line 17 of your 1040 tax form.
- The person is a U.S. citizen or resident or a resident of Canada or Mexico.
- You provided more than half of the person's total support for the year.
- The person does not have a gross income of more than $32,000/year.
- You do not have a gross income of more than $140,000/year.
- The person is a child who lives with you and is under the age of 19.
- The person is a child attending college who is under the age of 24 and still lives with you for more than half the year.

An important point is that you can include medical expenses that you paid for any person who meets these requirements — even if you cannot claim an exemption for that person on your tax return. To include these expenses, the person must have been your dependent either at the time the medical services were provided or at the time you paid the expenses.

For purposes of the medical and dental expenses deduction, a child of divorced or separated parents can be treated as a dependent of both parents. Under most circumstances, each parent can include the medical expenses they pay for the child, unless the child's exemption is being claimed under a multiple support agreement.

You can also deduct on your tax return medical expenses you paid for someone who would have qualified as your dependent except that the person didn't meet the gross income or joint tax return test; see www.irs.gov/taxtopics/tc502.html. You may deduct on your tax return qualified medical expenses you pay for yourself, your spouse, and your dependents, including a person you claim as a dependent under a multiple support agreement. If either parent claims a child as a dependent under the rules for divorced or separated parents, each parent may deduct on their tax return the medical expenses he or she actually pays for the child.

As with most government programs, certain rules and restrictions apply and may change frequently. Sometimes the IRS even offers a newer tax credit, so be sure to contact your accountant or the IRS at www.irs.gov for more information.

Is there any way around this restriction?
You may have the option of using a medical care reimbursement account through work, which, used effectively, may allow you to get around this restriction. With a reimbursement account, you pay your medical bills with pretax dollars, which has the same tax-saving impact as deducting every dollar that you pay. In 2003, the IRS ruled that the cost of nonprescription medicines can be paid with pretax reimbursement account money, even though such costs don't count toward the deduction.

What if I am self-employed?
If you are self-employed and have a net profit for the tax year (this also applies if you are a partner in a partnership or a shareholder in an S corporation) you may want to deduct your premiums and claim any supplementary healthcare expenses as a business expense instead of as a medical credit. As an adjustment to income, 100 percent of the amount you pay for medical insurance for yourself and your spouse and dependents is deductible on a Form 1040. You may not take this deduction for any month in which you or your spouse were eligible to participate in any subsidized health plan maintained by your employer or your spouse's employer.

The only time you can deduct more than 7.5 percent of your AGI is if you file Form 1040, U.S. Individual Income Tax Return, and itemize your deductions. Careful tax planning may allow you to take more medical deductions during one tax year instead of spreading them over two. For example, in a year in which you already have substantial medical expenses, schedule and pay for your routine doctor or dentist appointments by December 31 instead of early in the next year.

I have developed a condition that requires long-term care. Can I still use this deduction?
The costs of qualified long-term care services can generally be included as medical expenses. Deductible medical expenses also include a portion

(based on age of the insured) of the premiums paid for qualified long-term care insurance.

There is a health coverage tax credit available to certain individuals who receive a pension benefit referred to as Health Coverage Tax Credit (HCTC). This program pays 65 percent of qualified health plan premiums for eligible trade-impacted workers and certain Pension Benefit Guaranty Corporation (PBGC) benefit recipients throughout the year for those that qualify. To find out if you qualify, go to www.irs.gov or the PBGC website at www.pbgc.gov.

What defines these expenses?

Generally, unreimbursed medical and dental expenses include amounts paid for the diagnosis, cure, relief, treatment, or prevention of disease, and for treatments affecting any part or function of the body, but they must be primarily for the alleviation or prevention of a physical or mental defect or illness. You cannot include the cost of cosmetic surgery that is solely for the purpose of improving your appearance. Advance payments are not deductible until the service is rendered. Other expenses that may not be deducted include the following:

- Legal abortion
- Sterilization, such as a legal operation to prevent having children (such as a vasectomy)
- Acupuncture
- Inpatient treatment for alcoholism or drug rehabilitation programs (including transportation, meals, and lodging provided by the center)
- Air conditioner necessary for relief from allergies or other respiratory problems (less any increase in the value of your home resulting from installation of air conditioning)
- Clarinet and lessons to treat improper alignment of child's upper and lower teeth
- Swimming (the cost of therapeutic swimming prescribed by a physician)
- Stop-smoking programs
- Diet (when prescribed by a doctor, you can deduct the extra cost of purchasing special food to alleviate a special medical condition)
- Elastic hosiery for circulation problems

- Reclining chair bought on a doctor's advice by a person with a cardiac condition
- Ambulance service
- Artificial limbs and teeth
- Transplants of organs (not of hair)
- Chiropractic fees
- Christian Science practitioner fees
- Dental expenses
- Eyeglasses, contact lenses, hearing aids, dentures, crutches, wheelchairs, wheelchair lifts, wigs, and insulin needles
- Replacement of lost or damaged contact lenses
- Eye surgery (including surgery to correct vision)
- The purchase and care of a guide dog or another animal that aids the blind, deaf, or disabled
- Certain fertility enhancements (for details, please check www.irs.gov)
- Hospital expenses such as meals and lodging provided by a hospital during medical treatment
- Health insurance premiums not paid with pretax dollars
- Laboratory fees, exams, and x-rays
- Lead-based paint removal
- Legal fees needed to authorize treatment for mental illness
- The portion of life care or advance payment that you pay to a retirement home that is for medical care
- Lodging up to $50 per person per day (when necessary to receive medical care)
- Admission and transportation to a medical conference for a chronic illness of you, your spouse, or your dependent
- Fees paid to physicians, surgeons, specialists, dentists, psychologist, surgeons, chiropractors, acupuncturists, nurses, physiotherapists, speech therapists, audiologists, naturopaths, therapists, psychiatrists, psychologists, and other medical practitioners
- Medicines such as prescriptions, insulin, oxygen, and other required medical supplies
- Institutional care such as nursing homes and psychiatric hospitals, including nursing services

- Special education recommended by a doctor for learning disabilities caused by mental or physical impairment
- Telephone and television equipment and repair for a hearing impaired person
- Transportation expenses including bus, taxi, plane, or 22 cents per mile you drive for medical purposes plus parking fees and tolls (be sure to keep receipts and look up the deduction rates of these items for tax purposes at www.irs.gov)
- Weight loss program for a specific disease diagnosed by a physician (such as obesity, hypertension, or heart disease)
- Wheelchair purchase and repair
- Lifetime care advance payments
- Legal fees paid to authorize mental illness
- Qualified long-term care insurance contracts (subject to additional limitations such as age; these limitations can be found on www.irs.gov)
- Membership in an association that gives cooperative or so-called free-choice medical service, or group hospitalization and clinical care
- Social Security tax, Medicare tax, FUTA, and state employment tax for workers providing medical care

Certain special equipment installed in a home or for improvements that have a medical purpose (such as installing ramps in your home, widening doorways, and installing support bars) can also be included. However, only the amount of the expense that exceeds the increase in the property value of your home is deductible. Amounts paid to buy and install special plumbing fixtures for medical reasons in a home you rent are deductible if the landlord does not reimburse you or lower the rent to compensate.

Any special equipment or treatments you receive are also deductible. If you have a medical condition that can be helped by a sauna, a whirlpool, massage, or other type of treatment, it can come from someone other than a licensed physician, and would still be deductible. Be sure to obtain a written note from your doctor saying you need those services as proof for the IRS.

You *may not* deduct expenses for cosmetic surgery, dancing lessons, diaper service, funeral expenses, health club dues, maternity clothes, nonprescription drugs, nutritional supplements, teeth whitening, or veterinary fees. You may deduct cosmetic surgery if it's necessary to improve a deformity related to a congenital abnormality, an accident, or a disease.

You *may not* deduct expenses reimbursed to you, thus you may have to divide the cost of expenses equally according to who paid what, unless you can show otherwise.

To see some examples or get more information on medical deductions, go to www.wwwebtax.com, www.irs.gov/publications/p502/index.html, or www.irs.gov/pub/irs-pdf/p502.pdf or call 800-829-1040. IRS publications can also be ordered by calling 800-829-3676.

CHAPTER 6

HEALTH MAINTENANCE ORGANIZATIONS (HMOs)

A HEALTH MAINTENANCE ORGANIZATION, or HMO, is a type of group health insurance plan. This is the most common type of health insurance, and most health insurance companies provide an HMO option—even Medicare. It also tends to be the least expensive kind of health insurance, partly because the cost of your care is spread out among many members.

Most HMOs require you to stay within their network, which results in less paperwork but limits your choice of doctors. HMOs also focus on prevention, and many programs promote healthier life choices and better health.

If you belong to an HMO and need routine medical care, you will go to the HMO's clinic (also known as the network). This network provides its service through a group of doctors, medical personnel, and facilities that work directly for the HMO; however, as a general rule, your primary doctor must be your first step, as he or she prescribes your treatment and your referrals. Any medical care is done in the network's clinics by its doctors *only*, which is why it is equally as important to find a primary care doctor you are comfortable with as a location of a clinic where that doctor practices.

Every time you go to see an HMO doctor, for including routine checkups, you can expect to pay a small copayment. The clinics generally have many doctors available who will treat you for whatever you need. However, if you have a rare condition and require a specialist who is not in your network, you may have to pay a hefty price for that doctor. Until recently, few referrals for care outside of the system were given. It's common for quality doctors to refuse to join these plans because of poor compensation and limited referrals. This is not the best option for patients who have unusual medical needs.

When you join an HMO, you pay a premium (a fixed monthly fee). This entitles you to the use of the healthcare network that provides a variety of medical benefits. In addition to your monthly premium, there is typically also a copayment for each individual healthcare service offered. For example, when you visit a physician, you may be asked to pay $20 for a primary care physician office visit and $10 for any prescriptions. Some health insurance plans and some services charge nothing. The major drawback of any HMO policy is that no care received outside of the healthcare network is covered.

The only services that are covered by the HMO are those that you receive from a doctor or hospital that contracts with the HMO. In rare cases, the insurance plan may accept prior authorization for services deemed medically necessary and are not available by the plans definitions, in order to receive treatment out of your plan.

Some HMOs assign you a primary care provider, but others may instead ask you to choose a doctor in the network that you feel comfortable with. Again, you are required to use the plan's network of providers to receive any benefits and referrals are needed from your primary care provider to see a specialist. Keep in mind that the HMO pays its healthcare providers a set monthly fee regardless of the amount of services. Some doctors may even get a kickback by keeping their referrals down.

Usually, your choice of doctors and hospitals are limited to those on the list. The insurance company may have agreements with the HMO to provide your healthcare. However, exceptions may be made in emergencies or when medically necessary.

The range of healthcare services covered by HMOs varies, so it is important to compare available plans in your area. Your local state insurance department can help provide you with a list of HMOs in your area as well as general background information on which healthcare services are covered.

Advantages and Disadvantages of HMO Health Insurance

HMOs do not require claim forms for office visits or hospital stays. Instead, HMO members present a card, like a credit card, at the doctor's office or hospital. However, in an HMO you may have to wait longer for an appointment than some other forms of insurance.

Because the HMO health insurance company charges a fixed fee for your healthcare, it is in their interest to make sure you get basic healthcare for your medical problems before they become serious.

Although there may be a small copayment for each office visit, your total healthcare costs will likely be lower and more predictable in an HMO than with fee-for-service insurance.

Unfortunately, it can be difficult to get specialized care under an HMO plan since you must first obtain a network referral. Any healthcare cost from other providers, except in emergencies, is not covered; however, situations covered as emergency care are strictly limited.

Another common concern is whether you will have to keep switching doctors because of physicians leaving the plan. A way to avoid this is by asking the HMO for its "physician turnover rate." The National Committee for Quality Assurance (NCQA) may also be able to provide you with this information or at least a quality assurance record at 888-275-7585 or www.ncqa.org.

Is an HMO Right for Me?

Here is a list of questions to help guide your decision if an HMO is the right insurance for you. If the HMO cannot answer some of the following questions, you might want to reconsider:

- How many doctors can I choose from?
- Is the network made up of private or group practice physicians?
- Which doctors are accepting new patients?
- Can I change my primary care physician?
- What is the procedure for referrals to specialists?
- How easy is it to get an appointment?
- How far in advance must routine visits be scheduled?
- What arrangements are there for handling emergency care?

- What healthcare services are offered?
- Are there limits to medical tests, surgery, or other services?
- What happens if a special service is needed but not covered?
- Where are the hospitals that serve you located?
- What happens if I am out of town and need medical attention?
- What is the yearly total for monthly premiums?
- Are there any copayments? For which services and how much?

As stated previously, HMO premiums can vary considerably, even within the same state. The best way to save on your own payments is to compare as many plans and companies as possible.

You can get an instant health insurance quote from www.ehealthinsurance.com, or you can get information directly from a broker or a local agent, who will provide you with tailored premium quotes.

Although this may seem like the least expensive on paper, keep in mind that any sudden complications can make this type of plan very expensive. However, for people requiring mostly routine care, who have no unusual medical needs requiring out-of-network specialists and who like their medical care in an organized way, an HMO is a great choice.

CHAPTER 7

PPOs, POS, and FFS

Preferred Provider Organizations (PPOs) Give You Options

Preferred provider organizations (PPOs) are loosely organized groups of physicians and hospitals that have agreed to provide healthcare at predetermined levels of reimbursement for specific services. Unfortunately, the numbers of physicians and hospitals are generally limited, and. are often given standards to follow regarding the monitoring of utilization, what care is provided when, and the terms of the provision of care allowed under the arrangements.

You will have some flexibility with your healthcare decisions, especially when selecting your providers (both inside and outside the network). However, there is a definite financial incentive to remain within the network of PPO providers. for example, you will pay a higher percentage of the bill if you receive services from a hospital or doctor that is not part of the PPO network. Unlike HMOs, PPOs do not require you to have authorization to go to a doctor outside their plan. If you prefer a little more flexibility and a wider network of doctors to choose from, this may be the best choice for you. Keep in mind that PPOs may also vary slightly in their policies, so be sure to study each one carefully and ask them the questions listed later in this chapter.

In general, PPO insurance combines the lower cost of managed care with the greater degree of choice found in traditional health insurance. Similarly to an HMO, you will pay a fixed monthly premium. In return, the health insurance company and its healthcare network provide basic medical benefits to you.

Advantages and Disadvantages of PPOs

- Healthcare costs are relatively low when using the PPO networks
- You can consult any specialist, including ones outside the plan
- Seeing a primary care physician is not a prerequisite
- Paperwork is your responsibility if the care is nonnetwork
- Out-of-pocket costs per year are limited
- Cost of treatment outside of network is more expensive
- Copayments are larger than those of other managed care plans
- You may need to satisfy a deductible

PPO insurance is generally the most expensive managed care plan. Even if the premium quoted to you, for example, is comparable to that of an HMO, the extra fees associated with PPO insurance will increase its cost significantly. For example, coinsurance (lower charges if using network providers and higher charges if using nonnetwork providers). for preventive services, coinsurance is usually waived or replaced with a (low) copayment.

When you are out of the network, you will be responsible for a deductible before your PPO begins contributing. After your deductible is met, you will still be required to pay a percentage of the cost, and this percentage will be higher than if you had stayed in the network. You may also be required to pay the difference between what your out-of-network doctor charges and what your plan deems to be "reasonable and customary" for the service.

Is a PPO Right for Me?

If you are struggling with how to evaluate the quality of your PPO plan or want to know how an HMO compared to a PPO does servicewise, use the list of questions below as a guide. Again, if, for any reason, the health insurance policy does not answer to your satisfaction, be hesitant about purchasing it.

- How many doctors are there to choose from?
- Are doctors in the network private or group practice physicians?
- Where are the offices and hospitals in the network located?
- How are referrals to specialists handled?
- What hospitals are available through the plan?

- What arrangements does the plan have for emergency care?
- What healthcare services are covered?
- What preventive services are covered?
- Are there limits on medical treatments or other services?
- How much is the health insurance premium?
- Is there an out-of-pocket maximum?
- Is there a cap on services?
- Is there a financial cap?
- What, if any, are the copayments for specific services?
- How much more will it cost to use nonnetwork physicians?
- What is the deductible and coinsurance for nonnetwork care?

You should definitely determine what is required, what may be required, what financial considerations exist, and which health insurance options are best suited for all of these questions before purchasing a plan.

Point-of-Service (POS) Plans Offer Savings and Flexibility

A POS plan attempts to combine the freedom of a PPO with the lower costs of an HMO. In this plan, you will only pay a copayment or low coinsurance for contracted services within a network of preferred providers (for in-network care). However, like traditional fee-for-service insurance, you will have the flexibility to seek out-of-network care under the terms of traditional indemnity plans with a deductible, and a percentage coinsurance charge.

When you enroll in a POS plan, you are required to choose a primary care physician to monitor your healthcare. This primary care physician must be chosen from within the healthcare network, and becomes your point of service.

Your physician may then make referrals for you *outside* the network, the downside being that only limited compensation will be offered.

For medical visits within the healthcare network, your paperwork is completed automatically. However, if you go outside the network, it is your responsibility to fill out the forms, send bills in for payment, and keep an accurate account of your healthcare receipts.

Advantages and Disadvantages of POS Plans

With a POS plan:

- You have maximum freedom (for managed care).
- You are not limited to HMO network providers.
- For network care, copayments are low and there is no deductible.
- Annual out-of-pocket costs are limited.
- Ccopayments for nonnetwork care are high.
- There is a deductible for nonnetwork care.
- Getting referrals for specialists may be difficult.

The cost breakdown under a POS plan is similar to that of other managed care plans. It may be slightly less costly than a PPO because the health insurance company will still control most of your healthcare.

For example, to see a healthcare specialist you must first have a referral from your primary care physician. If the decision were up to you, you might choose an expensive nonnetwork specialist, but your primary care physician (who works within the network) will probably choose a specialist from within that network. These controls reduce the internal cost of the POS health insurance plan, which usually results in a lower premium for you.

Under a POS plan, you will pay a monthly premium and a copayment for all healthcare services covered under the plan and within the POS network. You'll also carry a deductible on any nonnetwork care, and after the deductible is met, you will pay a higher percentage of the remaining cost of care, and you may be required to pay the difference between what your out-of-network doctor charges and what your POS deems to be reasonable and customary.

Is a POS Plan Right for Me?

If, for any reason, a POS policy does not answer these questions to your satisfaction, please be hesitant about purchasing it.

- How many doctors are there to choose from?
- Are doctors in the network private or group practice physicians?
- Where are the offices and hospitals in the POS network located?
- How are referrals to specialists handled?
- What hospitals are available through the plan?
- What arrangements does the plan have for emergency care?

- What healthcare services are covered?
- What preventive services are covered?
- Are there limits on medical treatments or other services?
- How much is the health insurance premium?
- What, if any, are the copayments for specific services?
- How much more will it cost to use nonnetwork physicians?
- What is the deductible and coinsurance for nonnetwork care?
- Is there an out-of-pocket maximum?

Similar to the situation with an HMO, you are encouraged to participate in programs which will lead you to healthier choices and lifestyles. However, in a POS, you will have greater freedom to see out-of-network providers than with an HMO, but every time you do, it will cost extra. Your final decision about choosing this type of plan may rest on whether this additional freedom is worth the greater premium price.

Fee-For-Service (FFS) Plans

When you are a member of a fee-for-service (indemnity insurance) plan, your health providers are paid a fee for each service or supply provided. Their fees are billed at rates established by the plan.

Unlike HMOs, PPOs, or POS plans, fee-for-service is not a form of managed care. You may even receive reimbursement for your healthcare costs under a fee schedule. Your fees and reimbursements will be based on many factors, including the types of services provided, the geographic area of service, and office expenses of your doctor. It will also vary greatly from plan to plan.

The best part is that FFS offers you unlimited choice. You control your choice of physician and facility, from primary caregiver to specialist, surgeon, and hospital. Its flexible coverage also means immediate treatment for medical emergencies or unexpected illness.

However, FFS plans do have care restrictions. They do not traditionally cover preventive medicine, so checkups, office visits, and shots (as well as a few other services) will become your responsibility. This can make this impractical for a large family that requires a lot of routine visits and preventive care.

While it's hard to predict the annual cost of healthcare under an indemnity insurance plan, there are a few costs that come pretty standard:
- Monthly health insurance policy premium
- Yearly deductible before your health insurance begins to contribute
- Per visit coinsurance, or responsibility for a percentage of total expenses

As a rule, healthcare services not covered by your health insurance policy (such as checkups) also don't count toward satisfying your deductible. There are three kinds of indemnity insurance coverage:

Basic health insurance covers:
- Hospital room and board and hospital care
- Some hospital services and supplies, such as x-rays and medicine
- Surgery, whether performed in or out of the hospital
- Some doctor visits

Major medical insurance covers:
- Covers treatment for long, high-cost illnesses or injuries
- Covers both inpatient and outpatient expenses
- Tends to be expensive

Comprehensive insurance covers:
- Combines basic and major medical insurance
- Varies in price according to the level of coverage

CHAPTER 8

MEDICARE AND OTHER GOVERNMENT PROGRAMS

THERE ARE SEVERAL INEXPENSIVE and even free health-care programs offered by the government. They are available for the elderly and those who meet certain financial standards. Unfortunately, these programs are hard to find and difficult to understand.

If you don't understand something, continue calling until you do, or demand to speak to someone that understands the program and can explain it in a simpler way. Set aside a day to do your research. Read the following two chapters to learn the basics, and continue your search until you find a plan that works for you. Be prepared to stay on hold and be transferred several times. Take notes and get down names of people and their numbers.

The Railroad Retirement Board (RRB) replaces Social Security benefits for railroad employees, providing retirement pay as well as disability and survivor benefits. There are similar programs out there that are not advertised due to lack of advertising funds, being new, or (sometimes) the program not wanting to advertise because it is money out of their pocket if you qualify. As you inquire about programs along your search, be sure to ask if any new programs for healthcare benefits have been created, as you never know what you may find and what you qualify for. To find out more information about the Railroad Retirement Board program, go to www.rrb.gov or call 800-808-0772 to find out the nearest RRB office serving your area so you may speak with an RRB representative.

In brief, the most common government healthcare programs are:
- Medicare Plans A, B, and D
- Medicare Advantage plans (Part C)
- Private contracts
- Medigap
- Medicare and disability insurance
- Medicaid
- Program of All-Inclusive Care for the Elderly (PACE)
- Children's Health Insurance Program (CHIP)
- Department of Health
- Local chronic illness support groups
- TRICARE (military coverage, covered in Chapter 10)

Medicare

In early 2006, the prescription drug benefit (which I will discuss later) kicked in, and everyone covered by Medicare will have more choices to make. They will be eligible to:
- Stay in traditional Medicare, a Medicare HMO, or a retiree plan without signing up for the drug benefit
- Stay in traditional Medicare and enroll in a stand-alone drug plan or
- Enroll in a private health plan that offers drug coverage and Medicare health services.

In order to be eligible for Medicare, you must meet the following criteria:
- You must be 65 years old and you or your spouse must have worked for at least 10 years in Medicare-covered employment.
- You must have been a citizen or permanent resident of the United States for the five-year period proceeding the month of enrollment.
- If you are younger than 65, you might also qualify for coverage if you have a disability or have chronic kidney disease.

If you are still unclear about your Medicare eligibility, go to the following website to determine what Medicare benefits you are entitled to: www.medicare.gov/MedicareEligibility/home.asp.

If you are planning to enroll in Medicare, be sure to call Social Security at least three months before your 65th birthday to verify that you are properly enrolled in the Social Security system. Due to the constant changes in the national healthcare system, there is always a possibility of your information getting lost. The number of the Social Security office is 800-772-1213 or 800-325-0778 (TTY).

You cannot begin to receive Medicare benefits unless you are in the Social Security system. Once you are 65, you are also entitled to a "discounted" rate on Social Security benefits despite the retirement age being raised to 67.

Both Part A and Part B of Medicare are considered to be the original Medicare plans and your enrollment is needed in both of these plans if you want to join a Medicare Advantage plan (see page 96 for more information). Every November you are given the choice between the original Medicare program (fee-for-service program) and a Medicare Advantage plan. If you fail to make a selection but are already enrolled in one of the two options, you will simply remain in that plan for another year.

In other words, whether you are a new beneficiary investigating Medicare options, or an old beneficiary who needs more out of your Medicare benefits, September is a great time to mark your calendar to begin your research. By the time November comes around, you should have the information you need to join the correct Medicare plan.

Medicare Part A

Medicare Part A helps pay inpatient care in hospitals, including critical access hospitals, skilled nursing facilities and some home care and hospice care. It does not cover doctor visits, long-term care, prescription drugs, dental care, cosmetic surgery, routine foot care, glasses, or hearing aids. You may have to pay a monthly payment or premium, depending on your reason for acceptance into the Medicare system (such as age or disability). You may also qualify based on a spouse's or a parent's record, as well as the number of quarters that Medicare will cover.

These "quarters" are also known as Social Security "credits." As you work and pay taxes, you earn credits that count toward eligibility for future Social Security benefits. The maximum you can earn is four credits each year. Most people need 40 credits to qualify for benefits. Most workers earn more credits than needed in their lifetime of work to be eligible for Social Security. Extra credits will not increase your eventual Social Security benefits, but extra earned income may increase the benefit amount. Younger people need fewer credits to qualify for disability or for their spouse or children to qualify for survivors' benefits. A website that explains this is www.ssa.gov/pubs/10072.html.

Some other factors that may have an effect on having a premium are if you are already receiving retirement benefits from Social Security or the Railroad Retirement Board.

If you are under age 65, you can get Part A without having to pay a premium if:

- You have received Social Security or Railroad Retirement Board disability benefits for 24 months.
- You are a kidney dialysis or kidney transplant patient.

Medicare Part B

Medicare Part B helps cover doctors' services and outpatient care as well as other medical services that Part A does not cover (such as physical, occupational therapy, some home healthcare, ambulance transportation and a variety of tests and services).

You must pay a premium for Part B. The Part B monthly premium in 2005 was $78.20. This premium may be higher if you did not sign up for part B when you first became eligible, except in special circumstances. Check to see if those circumstances apply to you by going to this website: www.cms.gov.

There may also be a yearly deductible of $110, which is usually about 80 percent of the amount Medicare sets as the allowable charge for any service. This deductible increases annually. The premium is due to increase in 2007 for those individuals with annual incomes above $80,000, and couples with incomes above $160,000. These rates are set each December and can be checked by visiting www.medicare.gov or by calling 800-MEDICARE (800-633-4227). Depending on the state, it may subsidize part of the fee of low-income patients.

Medicare Part A Covers:

- **Inpatient hospital care:** Up to 90 days of hospital services each time you are admitted to the hospital, until you are out of the hospital or have not received skilled care in a nursing facility for 60 consecutive days. Also called a "benefit period."
- **Skilled care in a skilled nursing facility:** Up to 100 days of daily skilled nursing care, after a three-day prior hospitalization, in each benefit period. Please note that there is Medicare coverage after the 100th day in any one benefit period.
- **Home health care:** Medicare covers home health visits, if you are considered "homebound," (meaning it takes considerable effort for you to leave your home), you require skilled nursing services or skilled therapy services on an intermittent or part time basis, the services are provided by a Medicare certified home health agency, and your doctor has prepared a plan of care.
- **Hospice care:** Medicare will pay for an approved hospice program if a doctor certifies that the patient is terminally ill (is expected to live for less than six months). The patient chooses the hospice benefit, which is to care for the patient and his family rather than treating the illness, over the standard Medicare benefit.
- **Blood:** Pints of blood you receive at a hospital or skilled nursing facility during a covered stay. Under Part A, the patient pays for the first three pints of blood unless the patient or someone else donates blood to replace what the patient uses. However, there is a different policy for outpatient blood where the patient pays 20 percent above the three-pint deductible.

Please keep in mind that everything has guidelines. In addition, not every doctor accepts Medicare, so be sure your doctor participates in the program. If he or she does not, you may want to talk to someone in your State Health Insurance Assistance Program, listed online at http://hiicap.state.ny.us/ home/ link08.htm#links, as well as your doctor to see if he or she will opt to sign a private contract for healthcare benefits.

Medicare Part B Covers:

- Helps pay for doctors' and outpatient hospital services: including some preventative services such as bone mass measurements, cardiovascular screening blood tests, colorectal cancer screening, diabetes screening for people at risk for diabetes, glaucoma testing, Pap test and pelvic examinations (including a clinical breast exam), prostate cancer screening, screening mammograms, shots (vaccinations, including a flu shot once a season), and a one-time initial preventive physical exam within six months of when a person with Medicare first becomes enrolled in this plan.
- Physician services
- Rehabilitation therapy services: such as physical and occupational therapists
- Outpatient hospital services
- Ambulance services (when medically necessary)
- Diagnostic and laboratory tests: such as blood tests and urinalysis
- Mental health services
- Durable medical equipment such as prosthetic/orthotic items
- Chiropractic services
- Clinical trials
- Dental services
- Diabetic supplies
- Emergency services
- Eyeglasses, foot exams, hearing and balance exams
- Kidney dialysis services
- Medical nutrition therapy services
- Practitioner services
- Prescription drugs (except for certain cancer drugs)
- Surgical dressings
- Telemedicine (available in some rural areas)
- Tests (such as MRIs, x-rays, CT scans, EKGs, and some other diagnostics when medically necessary)
- Transplants
- Some emergency services in Mexico and Canada, as well as urgently needed care

Medicare Part D: Medicare Prescription Drug Benefits

Medicare Part D, formally known as the Medicare Prescription Drug Improvement and Modernization Act of 2003 (MMA) has been and probably will still be in process of deelopment long after this book is published.

As of January 2006, Medicare beneficiaries have the option of enrolling in either a new prescription drug plan (PDP) (fee-for-service) or a Medicare Advantage (MA) plan (formally known as Medicare Part C), which works like an HMO or regional PPO and covers drugs as well as other benefits.

In order to enroll, you must have already enrolled in Medicare Part A or B. You can be charged a late penalty, so make sure to enroll as soon as you are eligible. As in Part B, there is an additional monthly premium. HHS has estimated that those whose incomes exceed $11,500 will pay an average premium of $35 per month, depending on geographic location and choice of plan, in addition to a $250 deductible (these costs may vary depending on the plan you choose). The premium covers 25 percent of the cost of the standard drug benefit. For example, the standard drug benefit may be from the $250 deductible, 25 percent copayment up to $2,250 as long as the benefit package offered. This drug plan and costs may vary, largely due to its estimated value and its availability.

> *I am a grandmother of three who qualifies for Medicare Part D with monthly drug expenses of about $500. The first time I used my plan, I was asked to pay $312 (my $250 deductible, plus 25 percent due of the remaining $250). The next four months, I'm asked to pay $125 (25 percent of $500). When I reach my $2,850 cap in my sixth month, I have to pay 100 percent of my prescription drug costs—until my total costs reach $3,600. After $3,600 I only have to pay 5 percent of my drug costs. Luckily, I am able to plan ahead of time and save money throughout the year to provide for the months when I am expected to pay my full prescription costs.*
>
> *—Susan Greenspan, age 73*

On the other hand, those who qualify for special assistance (as determined by Medicare) may pay no premiums or deductibles, nor will they have a gap in their coverage. They will, however, be required to pay $2 for generics and $5 for brand names, but they will have no out-of-pocket expenses once their costs pass the $5,100 catastrophic limit. In order to see what Medicare drug plan you qualify for, you must call Medicare at 800-MEDICARE. Be sure to have the following information available:

- Your Medicare card number
- Your date of birth
- The effective date of your Medicare Plan A or Plan B
- The names of the prescriptions you are taking
- How many times a day you are taking these prescriptions and the dosage amount

If you have this information, the Medicare representative should be able to recommend you at least three Medicare drug plans that may be best for you as well as your premium, copay, deductible costs, and even the pharmacies in the network, as well as calculate how much you would pay for each drug on that plan.

You may also have to pay the full cost of your prescriptions through a second large deductible, called "the gap," which is 100 percent of your prescriptions from $2,280 until a $3,600 out-of-pocket spending cap is reached. Please remember that this out-of-pocket requirement does not include your premium payments, copayments, deductibles, and other costs, if they are paid for by another health plan. In order to calculate your out-of-pocket expenses of your prescription drug costs under the Medicare prescription drug law signed by President Bush in December 2003, go online to www.kaisernetwork.org/static/kncalc.cfm.

There is no definitive list of drugs or drug categories for Part D. Individual plans choose their own lists, and although the U.S. Pharmacopeia (USP) suggested guidelines, these are not required. Until the Part D plans are formally approved (which will not occur until at least September 2006), the USP suggested categories and classes are the only list, available at www.usp.org.

Once you join Medicare Part D, you are obligated to remain in the drug plan for a year, even if you develop a new medical problem. The downside to this is that the drug plans can change the drugs it cover sduring that year with only 60 days' notice and is not required to provide the information directly to you. In other words, if the FDA decides that it is going to pull a drug, it must notify your plan within 60 days of doing so. Unfortunately, it is up to you to make sure your drug is still on the market and find a substitute. As of now, the drugs that are not covered by most Medicare plans are the following:

- Benzodiazepines (tranquilizers), although some Medicare plans will pay for some of these drugs if you pay an extra premium.
- Barbiturates (sleeping pills)
- Medicines and cough medicines
- Vitamins or prenatal or fluoride prescriptions
- Anorexia, weight loss, or weight gain prescriptions
- Nonprescription drugs
- Cosmetic or hair growth prescriptions
- Fertility drugs
- Outpatient treatment when a drug is exclusive to a certain test, procedure, or service

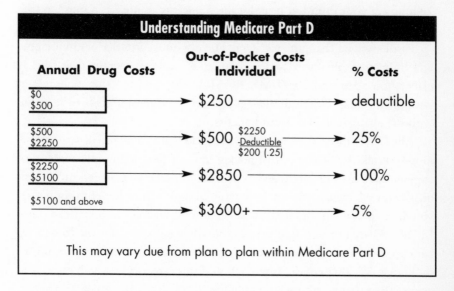

In addition, Medicaid may not pay for drugs that are covered under Medicare Part D but may assist for drugs that are not on the Medicare Part D's list.

If a drug that you have been using is pulled from your Medicare plan, you should follow these steps:

- Call your Medicare plan, and see what substitutes are available for that drug.

- If there is none available, or the substitutes are not adequate (as determined by your physician), or if there is a drug not on the list that is considered necessary to maintain or improve your health, call Medicare and ask for a formality exception. Typically, the formality exception form is filled out and a statement about your treatment is needed from your physician.
- Medicare may honor your request and waive the drug restrictions or require you to pay a higher level of coverage in order to continue or get treatment with that drug.

This same process will also take effect for a drug that is not offered on any plans in your area, if it is considered necessary by your primary physician for your treatment upon your initial enrollment. This is called an initial coverage determination or decision. Medicare is required to answer within 72 hours of your submission, and if the request is granted, it is good for the rest of the year.

Part D will be changing yet again. The discount cards that are in use now will be phased out by May 15, 2006, and another program may take its place. You can call 800-MEDICARE or go to the website at www.medicare.gov periodically (at least every three months) to keep up with the changes and the latest benefits.

After all of those costs, you may be curious if this plan will save seniors money at all. If you pay out of pocket, do not have many pharmaceutical expenses, and are not subsidized by any other insurance plan, it won't. If you qualify for Medicaid, you are better off taking its drug benefit program. If you have private insurance, try staying with that as well, at least until Medicare Part D irons itself out. Those who will save a lot on Part D are patients who have out-of-pocket pharmaceutical expenses that amount to more than $3,600 per year. If you fall into this category, you will pay 5 percent of the pharmaceutical amount and CMS will pay the other 95 percent.

Medicare Advantage Plans

If you have both Medicare Part A and Part B, you can enroll in a Medicare Advantage plan to cover your other medical expenses, including some prescription drugs. However, this applies only if it's included in the specific plan that serves your geographic region. If you move when enrolled, you may be offered the option of staying in the plan as long as you are moving to an area that still has access to all the basic benefits. Most plans are national, so it is likely that basic benefits will be covered. However, I suggest calling 800-MEDICARE to verify your benefits when you move. If they are not available, the Medicare representative should be able to find another plan that covers the benefits you need.

You may not be denied enrollment based upon your health status or certain other factors. If you have end-stage renal disease you can be excluded, but if you develop end-stage renal disease while enrolled in a Medicare Advantage plan, you cannot be required to leave the plan.

Previous to 2006, you were given the freedom to enroll in or leave Medicare Advantage plans at anytime. Now, however, there is a six-month lock-in for current members, and eventually you will be locked in to a Medicare Advantage plan for the entire year.

In the past, there have been many problems with Medicare Advantage plans and appeals, and many plans have pulled out of the Medicare market entirely. Err on the side of caution when enrolling. Be sure to read all details, especially any timelines and limitations before signing. Call Medicare at 800-MEDICARE, and be sure the representative can answer your questions completely and can send you written confirmation of the benefits and guidelines. Ask the Medicare representative the following questions:

- What coverage will be available under each plan in my geographic area?
- What plans will be offered, and what happens to my coverage if they do not remain in business?
- What options are available in the Medicare Advantage program that may be able to meet my needs (if they are not covered by the traditional Medicare plan)?
- What problems may develop within the appeal systems?
- If I am coming from a group plan, will I lose benefits once my group is divided into different plans?

The following Medicare Advantage Plans, formerly known as Medicare + Choice, are available in most parts of the country.

Coordinated Care Plans or Medicare Managed Care Plans

These plans include health maintenance organizations (HMOs), provider-sponsored organizations (PSOs), local preferred provider organizations (PPOs), and other network plans (except MSA and PFFS plans). Some plans serve only special populations, such as people in nursing homes or people who are covered by both Medicare and Medicaid.

These plans provide coverage for healthcare services, such as the ability to use in-plan or out-of-plan healthcare providers. Some will limit your choice of providers. Some plans may offer additional benefits for an extra premium. Some plans offer a combination of a limit on the choice of providers and supplemental benefits.

These plans are becoming extremely popular since they providee more options. In some cases, you may not even have to give up your old insurance plan but simply transfer to its Medicare benefits. Your option here is to call up the company or go to the Medicare website at www.medicare.gov and search the "Compare Health Plan Options in Your Area" option. If you already know what you already have, what you want, what is important to you, your zip code, and the price you are willing to pay for a premium, you can easily select the plan that best suits your needs.

Unfortunately, not all insurance companies are participating in Medicare benefits. Some are not accepting new members, and others require certain guidelines in order to apply. In order to find out more about these managed care plans or coordinated care plans, be sure to call 800-MEDICARE, and a representative should be able to explain the benefits of these plans and will take you through the selection process and find out which insurance companies are offering Medicare benefits in your community. For more detailed questions, you may have to call the individual company.

Medicare Private Fee-for-Service Plans

If you enroll in a fee-for-service plan, your doctor will be reimbursed at a rate determined by the plan, without referring to the Medicare Part B reasonable charge or limiting charge restrictions. Basically, you can see any provider as long as he or she is in the Medicare network of providers and will accept Medicare's payment for services provided. The rates set by these plans may be substantially higher than those in the traditional Medicare program.

Private fee-for-service plans are required to provide you with explanations of their benefits and liabilities. The plans are also required to provide you with advanced balance billing information before you incur expenses for inpatient care. In order to avoid any surprises, you may want to get a complete list of services/procedures your doctor wishes to perform and submit it to the MA plan in order to map out what is covered and not covered, and then negotiate the rest with your provider.

Medical Savings Account (MSA) Plans

These plans combine a health insurance plan carrying a high deductible with a medical savings account. Medicare MSA started as an option designed to test whether MSAs would give both you and the Medicare program better control over healthcare spending.

In a Medicare MSA plan, Medicare pays the premium and makes deposits to the MSA you establish. Unlike other Medicare health plans, there are no limits on what providers can charge you above the amount paid by your Medicare MSA plan. You use the money deposited in your Medicare MSA to pay for your medical expenses. If you don't use all the money, next year's deposit will be added to your balance.

Money can be withdrawn from a Medicare MSA for nonmedical expenses, but that money will be taxed. If you enroll, you must stay in the program for a full year. You can sign up only in November of each year or during special enrollment periods. If you use all your Medicare MSA money, you are responsible for paying all of your medical expenses until you meet the deductible for your plan. This deductible can be considerably higher than those of other Medicare health plans.

Medicare Advantage organizations offering MSA plans are not permitted to offer prescription drug coverage, other than those expressly required by Parts A and B. Basically whatever the original Medicare plans offer in terms of prescription drugs is what the MSA plan offers and it is not required to offer anything else. As of the publication of this book, no Medicare Advantage organization has offered an MSA and high deductible plan—but it may be offered eventually. You should inquire if this is an interest. If you are enrolled in a MSA plan, you must remain in that plan for a year, although if this is your first year in the plan, you will have until the December 15th after your enrollment to leave the program.

In general, coverage is offered for most hospital services, as well as for other services with substantial balances due.

Medicare Specialty Plans

These plans are designed to give you all your Medicare healthcare, as well as more focused care to manage a disease or condition in an efficient, effective, high-quality manner. The Religious Fraternal Benefit (RFB) Society plans and private contracts described below are examples of these types of plans.

Religious Fraternal Benefit (RFB) Society Plans

Some Medicare Advantage plans may be offered by religious and fraternal organizations. These organizations can restrict enrollment to their members. The plans must meet Medicare financial solvency requirements, and Medicare may adjust payment amounts to the plans to meet the characteristics of the individuals enrolled. RFB Society plans may be any type of Medicare Advantage plan. To find out if there is an RFB Medicare plan in your area, call Medicare at 1-800-MEDICARE or go to its website at www.cms.gov.

Private Contracts

You may also enter into an agreement with certain providers that will offer you a private contract. These contracts are outside the Medicare program, and no Medicare payments will be made under these arrangements. You would be required to pay all the costs in accordance with your private contract. In addition, your provider must agree (in writing) not to bill Medicare for *any* services for a period of two years.

Your provider will warn you that the Medicare limits on balance billing will not apply under this option and that Medicare supplemental insurance (Medigap) policies may not pay benefits on your claims. The contract should also make clear that you *may* seek medical care from other healthcare providers who have not entered into private contracts and who are, therefore, permitted to bill Medicare.

For help comparing these health plan choices, compare Medicare Prescription Drug Plans at www.medicare.gov or call 800-633-4227. Before you call or go to the website, be sure you know the answers to the following questions:

- Are you over 65?
- Do you have other health insurance coverage?
- Do you have Medicare Part A and/or Part B?
- What is your zip code?

When you use the finder, you will get a personal summary page either immediately or within three weeks by mail (your selection). This information will provide you with the information you need to compare plans in your area.

If you have questions about your eligibility for Medicare Part A or Part B, or if you want to apply for Medicare, you should call the Social Security Administration at 800-772-1213. You can also get information from this number about purchasing Part A as well as Part B, even if you do not qualify for premium-free Part A.

Keep in mind that your choices may vary if you are enrolled in Medicaid, have employer or union coverage, veterans or military retiree benefits, or have end-stage renal disease (permanent kidney failure).

Medigap

Medigap is a health insurance policy sold by private insurance companies to fill the "gaps" in the original Medicare plan. Medigap policies help you pay some of the healthcare costs that the original Medicare plan doesn't cover. If you are in the original Medicare plan and have a Medigap policy, Medicare will pay its share and your Medigap policy will pay its share of your healthcare costs.

Currently, there are ten standardized Medigap plans, called "A" through "J." Medigap policies must follow federal and state laws that are designed to protect you. Unfortunately, Medigap policies with drug benefits were no longer offered as of January 1, 2006. Medigap does not cover the following:

- Long-term care to help you bathe, dress, eat, or use the bathroom
- Vision or dental care
- Hearing aids
- Private-duty nursing
- Prescription drugs

The following website will help you decide if Medigap is necessary to help cover your healthcare needs: www.medicare.gov/mg compare/home.asp.

Appeals

No matter which plan you are interested in, before committing, please be sure to investigate the appeals process. Recently, Medicare contractors were given twice as much time to review appeals at the contractor level. To find out your Medicare rights as well as answer other questions about the Medicare system, check out: www.medicarerights.org.

Medicare and Disability

You can receive Medicare benefits if you are deemed disabled by Social Security—no matter what age you are. Medicare benefits kick in after two years of receiving disability benefits from Social Security, regardless of the nature of your disability. The only exception is amyotrophic lateral sclerosis (Lou Gehrig's disease). If you have this disease, you do not have the 24-month waiting period. Individuals who qualify for Medicare because of a disability have exactly the same coverage as those who qualify because of age. To find out more information, go to the website at www.social security.gov or call 800-772-1213.

State Health Departments

States are allocated federal funds, and they have the ability to grant those funds to different medical programs throughout the state. To find out if you qualify for one of these medical programs, you can locate your state health department by going to www.cdc.gov/doc.do/id/0900f3ec80226c7a. Every state should have a health department number listed that you can call and inquire about new as well as renewed state healthcare programs. Remember to be specific and patient; it may take a few calls before you are directed to someone who actually knows what the state offers.

CHAPTER 9

MEDICAID

M EDICAID IS A JOINT FEDERAL and state program that helps with the medical expenses of some people with low incomes and limited resources. These programs vary from state to state because of the broad guidelines set by the federal government, which are:

- Each state establishes its own eligibility criteria.
- Each state sets its own rate of payment for services.
- Each state determines the type, duration, amount, and scope of services.
- Each state administers its own program.
- To be eligible for Medicaid, you must be one of the following:
  - A pregnant woman or have a child or children under the age of 6 whose family income is below 133 percent of the poverty guideline
  - A member of a low-income family who meets the State's Temporary Assistance for Needy Families (TANF) requirements or on welfare
  - Receiving supplemental security income (SSI)
  - A recipient of adoption or foster care assistance
  - Aged, blind, or disabled

Few states cover single, healthy adults. If your state does, you will also be required to meet state income and resource standards, as well as certain other requirements, such as being a resident of the state and a U.S. citizen or qualified immigrant. Legal immigrants may also qualify under certain circumstances, depending on their date of entry into the country. Illegal aliens do not qualify, except for emergency care.

Even if your income is above the definition of that of a low-income family, you may still be eligible for special Medicaid assistance. Check to see if you qualify by locating your local Medicaid office at www.cms.hhs.gov/ Telemedicine/03_StateProfiles.asp#TopOfPage or clicking on your state's name at www.statehealthfacts.org/cgi-bin/healthfacts.cgi. It will be listed under the state Health Department or the Department of Human Services. The names of programs change frequently, as do department names, so this may take some research, depending on your state of residence. A quick way to find some contacts is to go to your local hospital's social workers' department. Social workers are familiar with the top Medicaid programs but may not be as familiar with the more obscure programs. However, they should know who else to contact about other programs funded under Medicaid.

Finding a Program That Is Right for You

Once you find the correct number for the program you are interested in, write it down. Numbers rarely change, but program names often do. For example, D.C. Medicaid has a program called Medicaid "Spend-Down," which is also offered in 34 other states in the United States, but under many different names

In general, Medicaid services include the following:
- Inpatient hospital services
- Outpatient hospital services
- Prenatal care
- Vaccines for children
- Physician services
- Nursing facility services for aged persons
- Family planning services and supplies
- Rural health clinic services
- Home healthcare for persons who are eligible for skilled nursing services
- Laboratory and x-ray services
- Pediatric and family nurse practitioner services
- Nurse-midwife services
- Federally qualified health center (FQHC) services and ambulatory services of an FQHC that would be available in other settings
- Early and periodic screening, diagnostic, and treatment (EPSDT) services for children under the age of 21

Similarly to Medicare, Medicaid has many different insurance plans that are worth inquiring into, but the plans vary from state to state and have very distinct healthcare goals. Many of these plans cover routine medical, dental, and prescription expenses, and even emergencies. Ask about the various insurance plans when you speak to your local Medicaid representative.

Title 19 Eligibility

If you are a Medicare recipient, you may also be eligible for what is known as Title 19 under Medicaid. This is a medical assistance program for low-income people who are 65 years and older, disabled, or blind, or who meet some other category of eligibility. Some people have so little income that they automatically qualify for Medicaid. However, if you are a senior or have a disability, even if your income exceeds the income limit you can still qualify for Medicaid if you have medical bills that are equal to or greater than your "excess" income. The process of subtracting those medical bills from the individual's income over a six-month period is called a Medicaid "spend-down."

> *Recently, I had a medical bill of over $40,000 due to a hip fracture I incurred over the past year, and my healthcare insurance barely covered 50 percent of my hospital bill. Unfortunately, my monthly net income is only $715 per month, which put me over the $692 poverty level that I need to qualify for my state Medicaid. I panicked and called my local department of health, which put me in touch with a local social service representative. To my surprise, I was able to receive Medicaid due to the fact that my medical bills over that six-month period exceeded my income!*
>
> *—Amy Sullo, age 63*

In some states, seniors placed on spend-downs by their state Department of Social Services (DSS) have incomes that are in excess of the Medicaid limit set by DSS. You must ask you DSS what that limit is because it varies from state to state and tends to change annually. If your medical expenses equal or exceed your Medicaid limit, you will receive full Medicaid coverage—but only until the end of the six-month spend-down period. At that point, your situation will be reviewed again. Your state's DSS should be able to tell you if you are eligible for this program. You can find contact numbers for DSS here by looking it up in your local phone book or by searching for your state's department of social services.

The spend-down process is required for eligible seniors who live in their own homes, apartments, senior housing, or congregate housing, if they have income over the Medicaid limit. On the other hand, if you live in an institution such as a nursing home or a hospital, or in a residential care home, you do not have to go through the spend-down process, but it's you will have to contribute most of your income to the cost of your care.

If you are a recipient of state supplemental benefits or other home care programs for the elderly, you may not have to spend down your excess income. Medicaid is automatically provided with some of these programs.

In most cases, only medical bills for certain physician's services; hospital and prescription bills; medical supplies, such as bandages, gauze, and other items; over-the-counter drugs and vitamins prescribed by your doctor; and health insurance premiums, co-payments and deductibles are covered by some Medicaid programs. These payments are owed to you (and to your spouse, if your spouse's income was counted) if no other insurance or program will pay for them. (Some programs have exemptions for prescription drugs.) When applying for Title 19, there are limits on the bills that you have received before your application that you may use.

For more information, contact the nearest Area Agency on Aging on www.n4a.org or locate your local state department of social services.

Optional Medicaid Services

Other local Medicaid programs that may be able to help you might include federal matching funds. These would provide you with optional services different from more specific insurance plans. The following are the most common of the 34 currently approved optional Medicaid services:

- Diagnostic services
- Clinic services
- Intermediate care facilities for the mentally retarded (ICFs/MR)
- Prescribed drugs and prosthetic devices
- Optometrist services and eyeglasses
- Nursing facility services for children under the age of 21
- Transportation services
- Rehabilitation and physical therapy services
- Home and community-based care to certain persons with chronic impairments

Some states provide their residents with free services, for example, under the Breast and Cervical Cancer Prevention and Treatment Act (BCCPTA) of 2000, which helps state Medicaid programs to provide medical services to women diagnosed with breast or cervical cancer. In order for you to be eligible for Medicaid under this option, you must:

- Have been screened for and found to have breast or cervical cancer, including precancerous conditions, through the National Breast and Cervical Cancer Early Detection Program (NBCCEDP)
- Be under age 65
- Be uninsured and/or not eligible for Medicaid

For more information on this program, which is administered by the Centers for Disease Control and Prevention (CDC) under Medicaid, go to http://bphc.hrsa.gov or to www.cdc.gov to find out about other healthcare programs that may become available. You may also wish to call the CDC at 800-232-4636 between the hours of 8 A.M. and 4:30 P.M. EST.

Many Medicaid health services are available to those whot qualify. You may be surprised by the programs you qualify for. Unfortunately, there's no easy way to learn what will work for you; you will have to do some research and ask the right questions to questions.

Program of All Inclusive Care for the Elderly (PACE)

PACE programs provide preventive, primary, acute, and long-term-care services with the goal of allowing older individuals to continue living in their communities. It's an optional benefit under both Medicare and Medicaid that focuses entirely upon the elderly, if you are frail enough to meet your state's standards for nursing home care.

PACE features comprehensive medical and social services that can be provided in an adult day health center, home, or an inpatient facility. For most people, the service package provides the flexibility needed to continue living at home while receiving medical services, instead of having to take the more drastic step of being institutionalized. A team of doctors, nurses, and other health professionals will assess your needs, develop care plans, and deliver all your services, which are integrated into a complete healthcare plan. PACE is not offered in all states, only those that have chosen to offer PACE under Medicaid.

In order to be eligible, you must:
- Be at least 55 years of age
- Live in a PACE service area
- Be screened by a team of doctors, nurses, and other health professionals
- Sign and agree to the terms of the enrollment agreement

PACE services include all Medicare and Medicaid services provided by your state as well as 16 additional services, including social work, drugs, and nursing facility care. There are certain minimum services that PACE must provide, including:
- Primary care services
- Social services
- Restorative therapies
- Personal care and supportive services
- Nutritional counseling
- Recreational therapy

If you are also enrolled in adult day care services, your meals and transportation for those days are also covered. PACE services are available 24 hours a day, seven days a week, 365 days a year.

Generally, these services are provided in an adult day care health center setting, but occasionally include in-home and other referral services that enrollees may need. This includes such services as:
- Medical specialists
- Laboratory and other diagnostic services
- Hospital and nursing home care

Your degree of need is determined by PACE's medical team of care providers. These teams include:
- Primary care physicians and nurses
- Physical, occupational, and recreational therapists
- Social workers
- Personal care attendants
- Dietitians
- Drivers

This team usually has daily contact with you, allowing them to detect subtle changes in your condition and quickly react to changing medical, functional, and psychosocial problems.

PACE receives a fixed monthly payment per member enrolled from Medicare and Medicaid. The amount it receives remains the same during the entire contract year, regardless of the services you may need.

If you are enrolled in PACE, depending on your eligibility for Medicare and Medicaid, you may be required to pay a monthly premium. A list of PACE sites can be found on www.medicare.gov/Nursing/Alternatives/PaceSites.asp. To find out more information about the PACE program, call 703-535-1565 or go to the national PACE website at www.npaonline.org.

Children's Health Insurance Program (CHIP)

CHIP is a national program designed for families who earn too much money to qualify for Medicaid yet who cannot afford private health insurance for their children. Because it is associated with the state's Medicaid program, it may be confusing because the qualifiers and benefits are different. In order to qualify, the following criteria must be met:
- The child must be under 19 (some states include pregnant women).
- The family or child must not be eligible for Medicaid coverage.
- The parents must be U.S. citizens or legal immigrants; however, in certain states, there is a roster of "undocumented children" waiting to be put on a similar program called the Multi-National Unit.
- The family's income must be below 200 percent of the federal poverty level (this level may vary from state to state)

Depending on the exact program in CHIP that you register for, as well as your state, CHIP may cover:
- Immunizations
- Doctor's visits
- Prescription drugs
- Laboratory and diagnostic tests
- Well-child programs
- Prenatal care
- Hospitalizations
- Dental services
- Other medical services

Depending on where you live, you may be charged a small monthly premium based on your income. Sometimes CHIP is free (such as the program in Washington, D.C., called "DC Healthy Families"). To learn more about your child's eligibility and how to enroll, call 877-543-7669. You may also look up your state's medical assistance regional office at www.insurekidsnow.gov under "SCHIP State Map," or call your local department of Human Services or the Department of Health. Be sure to inquire about other programs your state may offer that may be available to your children, especially if they have more specific medical needs.

Department of Health

Each state's Department of Health offers several healthcare programs to those who do not qualify for either Medicare or Medicaid. Most of these programs cover routine dental, medical, prescription, and emergency care. Call your local Department of Health and ask to speak with someone who is familiar with the state's various medical assistance programs. You can easily locate your Department of health by checking your local phonebook. An example of this type of program is the DC Healthcare Alliance, which is funded by the D.C. government. It provides D.C. residents, both uninsured individuals and families, an opportunity for better healthcare. The DC Healthcare Alliance has the beneficiary work with a primary care provider and has access to preventive care. The program covers medical exams, dental exams, and eye exams. For more information, you can go to the website at www.chartered-health.com/Alliance.htm or call the Alliance at 202-842-2810.

Local Chronic Disease Support Groups

We all know that if you or a loved one has a chronic disease, it can be devastating both emotionally and financially. That is why these support groups are formed, to lobby for your interests, whether they be lower treatment costs, finding the least expensive insurance plan, or dealing with medical bills. Many people overlook the opportunity these local support groups offer when it comes to the financial side of these conditions. Most of the time, these groups are public or nonprofit, which means they are receiving grant money of some sort from a local or federal agency to help support people who have a certain chronic condition. In order to get an accurate list of these support groups, it is better if you know what disease you are inquiring about. When you have accurately diagnosed the disease, you can search the disease at the Centers for Disease and Prevention online at www.cdc.gov or call 800-311-3435 (press 0). Be sure to ask for your state health department's contact information. One you locate your state health department on the list, call it and ask for a list of the support groups in your area that pertain to your condition. An example of this list is in the appendix of this book. Please keep in mind that the Centers for Disease and Prevention may have created a more updated, concise list since this book was published.

Healthcare for Your Children

Medicaid, described earlier, has a special allotment of funds for children and their families who may be financially unable to afford health insurance even if they are employed. Every state has a different set of rules, but most states require the family to have at least one child under the age of 19 and an income of no greater than $32,000 a year for a family of four. Again, each state has a different set of rules. You can find out your state's rules by calling 877-543-7669.

Medicaid pays for doctors' visits, immunizations, hospitalizations, and emergency visits at little or no cost. Refer to the information on Medicare and Medicaid for the contact information for the program in your state.

Families who earn too much to qualify for Medicaid may be able to qualify for the State Children's Health Insurance Program (SCHIP). SCHIP was designed as a federal/state partnership, similar to Medicaid, with the goal of expanding health insurance to children whose families earn too much to be eligible for Medicaid but not enough to purchase private insurance, and to address the growing number of children without insurance.

SCHIP is designed to provide coverage to any children residing in a family with an income level 200 percent below the federal poverty level (FPL) or with an income 50 percent higher than the state's Medicaid eligibility threshold. State Medicaid is set by individual states. For example, the 200 percent in Virginia in 2006 is totaled at $2767 gross for family of 3 per month. This amount may change every year, but you will need to contact your state Medicaid office to find out the exact amounts. Some states have expanded SCHIP eligibility beyond the 200 percent FPL limit, and others cover entire families, not just children.

Unfortunately, not all children of low-income families are eligible. Some of the ineligible groups include:

- Children who are covered by a group health plan or health insurance
- Children who are members of a family that is eligible for state employee insurance based on employment with a public agency
- Children who are residing in an institution for mental diseases
- Children who are eligible for Medicaid coverage

If a state elects to establish an expanded Medicaid program using SCHIP, the eligibility rules of Medicaid apply.

Under the SCHIP program, the state has three options on how to structure its SCHIPP program. It may:

- Use SCHIP funds to expand Medicaid eligibility to children who previously did not qualify for the program
- Design a separate children's health insurance program entirely separate from Medicaid or
- Combine the Medicaid and separate program options

The SCHIP program varies among states depending on the option each state prefers to implement. The state may choose to care for only a child if he or she is under 18, the entire family including the child, or even a pregnant women. If a state opts for a separate child health program, certain other rules can affect eligibility:

- States may allow for self-declaration of citizenship.
- States are prohibited from enforcing duration-of-residency requirements.
- States may not enact lifetime caps or other time limits for eligibility.
- States may offer children 12 continuous months of eligibility;
- States may enforce enrollment caps and waiting lists for coverage, if these provisions are in the approved state plan.

When screening and enrolling children for SCHIP, states must establish a system to determine if a child is Medicaid eligible and provide a mechanism for enrollment in Medicaid if appropriate. States may also allow for a period of presumptive eligibility while the application and eligibility process is under way. Similarly to every other state plan, the SCHIP plan is constantly changing and adding and taking away programs, so it is always beneficial to check the SCHIP website and contact your appropriate state for more information at www.cms.hhs.gov/LowCostHealthInsFamChild to get the latest program updates.

Certain other programs that do not have as strict financial ability rules and cater to children who are simply uninsured. The following websites provide screening tools to help you determine if you are eligible for a variety of governmental programs: www.govbenefits.gov and www.benefitscheckup.org.

If searching for the right healthcare program for your child/children seems too difficult, some organizations have recently been formed to help assist you to find the best healthcare program for your uninsured child. One such program is called Covering Kids & Families (CKF).

As of 2005, CKF operated through statewide projects in 45 states and the District of Columbia and more than 140 local community projects. In addition, five states have CKF liaison grants that provide opportunities to participate in the national CKF initiative to help reduce the number of uninsured children in the United States who may not be eligible to enroll in Medicaid or SCHIFF. CKF does this by:

- Conducting and coordinating outreach programs
- Simplifying enrollment and the renewal processes
- Coordinating existing healthcare coverage programs

You can find out more about the program nearest you by calling 800-KIDSNOW or going to the website at http://coveringkidsandfamilies.org/projects/ to find out about the newest projects taking place in your state.

Some states, such as Florida, have a program such as KidCare, a health insurance program for uninsured children under age 19. Florida's program, for example, is made up of four parts: MediKids (www.floridakidcare.org); Healthy Kids (www.healthykids.org); the Children's Medical Services (CMS) Network (www.cms-kids.com), for children with special healthcare needs; and Medicaid for children (www.dcf.state.fl.us/ess). When you apply for the insurance, Florida's KidCare will determine which program your child is eligible for, based on age and family income.

An application is valid for 120 days after Florida KidCare receives it. If your children are not enrolled in MediKids, Healthy Kids, or the Children's Medical Services Network within the 120 days, Florida KidCare will notify you and you will need to reapply. An application that is older than 120 days may still be used to determine if your children are eligible for Medicaid.

Some Florida KidCare programs have limited space, and applications are accepted on a first-come, first-served basis. When MediKids, Healthy Kids, and the Children's Medical Services Network are full, enrollment for these programs closes. Medicaid, however, is always open to children who qualify.

If enrollment for MediKids, Healthy Kids, and the Children's Medical Services Network is closed, Florida KidCare will determine if your children are eligible for Medicaid. You will receive more information if your children are eligible for Medicaid. If your children are not eligible for Medicaid, you will need to reapply when MediKids, Healthy Kids, or the Children's Medical Services Network are open again.

Another example of a healthcare program for uninsured children is DC Healthy Families (see above), which is supported by the D.C. Department of Health, the Medical Assistance Administration, the Department of Human Services, the District of Columbia, the federal government, the Income Maintenance Administration, the Office of Maternal and Child Health, and the outreach contractor Houston Associates, Inc.

Again, some states include the whole family in the equation; others do not. DC Healthy Families covers children, adolescents under age 19 who live alone, pregnant women, and parents or guardians.

The benefits include:
- Doctor visits
- Immunizations (shots)
- School physicals
- Emergency care
- Hospital stays
- Prescription medicines
- Prenatal care
- Labor and delivery
- Vision care and glasses
- Dental care
- Family planning
- Transportation to doctor appointments
- Home healthcare
- Durable medical equipment

- Health education services
- Mental health services
- Drug and alcohol treatment

Benefits vary depending on the program you are enrolled in under DC Healthy Families. The three types of health plans are Amerigroup Corporation, DC Chartered Health Plan, and Health Right. More information about these programs and the varying benefits and qualification may be found by calling 202-727-1000 or at http://doh.dc.gov/doh/site/default.asp.

Every state has its own set of rules, and the above is an example of a program that may or may not be duplicated in another state. The only way to find out which program is best for your circumstances and your child is by investigating and going through some of the websites listed in this chapter, which may lead you to others.

CHAPTER 10

COVERAGE FOR THE MILITARY

THERE ARE TWO MAJOR TYPES of health insurance available for the military. The first is TRICARE, a managed healthcare system for active members of the U.S. military and their dependents. The second is the Department of Veterans Affairs (VA) health system, which gives benefits to eligible veterans of the U.S. armed forces. A managed healthcare system is any system of health payment or delivery arrangements whereby the health plan attempts to control or coordinate the use of health services by its enrolled members in order to contain health expenditures, improve quality, or both. Arrangements often involve a defined delivery system of providers with some form of contractual arrangement with the plan such as a health maintenance organization (HMO), which will be described later in the book.

TRICARE

TRICARE is the Department of Defense's worldwide healthcare program for active duty and retired uniformed services members and their families. If you're trying to find out if you are eligible, you should check your enrollment in the Defense Enrollment Eligibility Reporting System (DEERS).

The DEERS record will indicate the dates of eligibility. As long as you are active (in other words, putting on a uniform five days a week or more), you are eligible. You can also be eligible after being active for at least 20 years. It's your job, whether active, reserve, or retired, to ensure your family status (marriage, death, divorce, new child, and other information) and residential addresses are current in DEERS at all times. Eligibility confusion arises with military families. For example, if you are married to someone who receives TRICARE, be sure you are in the system by contacting DEERS. At times you might find that your benefits were not reimbursed even when your spouse was in the DEERS system. This is common, and most of the time the cause of it is that the provider submitted your Social Security number as the primary beneficiary instead of that of your spouse, who is the "military person" in the family. This is why it is important to not only get a breakdown of your medical bills before you leave the doctor's office, but to be sure your DEERS enrollment and updates are completed at uniformed services personnel offices, not TRICARE service centers. For more information about DEERS, contact the Defense Manpower Data Center Support Office (DSO) Telephone Center from 6 A.M. to 5 P.M. Pacific time, Monday through Friday, at the following toll-free number: 800-538-9552.

Once you have determined that you are in the DEERS system, you should identify the type of plan your region offers. There are three major regions in the United States with varying benefits; the West, North, and South. To locate the region you are in and find out more detailed information, go to www.tricare.osd.mil or www.tricare.osd.mil/factsheets/viewfactsheet.cfm?id=92.

There are several subplans in TRICARE:
- **TRICARE Prime,** a managed care option
- **TRICARE Extra,** a preferred provider option
- **TRICARE Standard,** a fee-for-service option
- **TRICARE for Life,** available for Medicare-eligible beneficiaries 65 and over
- **TRICARE Plus,** coverage for those who are supporting parents and/or grandparents; this option can also be economically linked
- **TRICARE Reserve Select (TRS),** continued care for reservists only
- **Extended Care Health Option (ECHO),** for active-duty family members with disabilities

TRICARE Prime

TRICARE Prime is a managed care option similar to a civilian health maintenance organization (HMO). Active duty service members are required to enroll in Prime.

Compared to other TRICARE options, Prime offers:
- The lowest out-of-pocket costs
- Active-duty members and their families pay no enrollment fees, annual deductibles, or copayments for care within the TRICARE network
- Retired service members have a $230 individual annual enrollment fee or a $460 family annual enrollment fee
- Minimal copays apply for care in the TRICARE network for pharmaceuticals, point-of-service (POS) and services under the Program for Persons with Disabilities (PFPWD). More information can be found at: www.mytricare.com/Internet/tric/tri/tricare.nsf/PGS/TRCRBscs_Prgrms_11. Active-duty family members do not pay copayments
- Most care is by military providers or civilian providers who belong to the TRICARE Prime network

Once you are enrolled, you are assigned a primary care manager (PCM) who will manage your care and will provide referrals for specialty care if needed. All referrals for specialty care must be arranged by the PCM to avoid additional charges. One of the best things about TRICARE Prime is that you are guaranteed certain access standards for care such as wait times, which are not offered by many other insurance plans outside of the military.

Active-duty family members, as well as retirees and their family members, are encouraged, but not required, to enroll in Prime. However, to receive the TRICARE Prime benefit, you must reside where TRICARE Prime is offered. To find out if it is in your area, ask your local TRICARE service center (TSC). You can find out the correct person to speak to by going to www.tricare.osd.mil/factsheets/viewfactsheet.cfm?id=92. If you are stationed in a remote area, TPR/TRICARE Prime Remote for Active Duty Family Members (TPRADFM) may be the option available to you and your family members.

TRICARE Extra and TRICARE Standard

TRICARE Extra and TRICARE Standard are available for all TRICARE-eligible beneficiaries who elect or are not able to enroll in TRICARE Prime. However, active duty service members are not eligible for Extra or Standard, because they are required to sign up for TRICARE Prime.

Both TRICARE Extra and Standard have the following advantages:
- No enrollment is required.
- There are no annual enrollment fees.
- There are no enrollment forms.
- Beneficiaries are responsible for annual deductibles, the total amount of covered medical expenses that must be paid by the patient before the insurance company begins paying benefits and cost shares, the amount the plan covers after the deductibles are met, are defined at http://tricare.osd.mil/TRICAREStandard/std-req.cfm. For example, if the patient chooses to have a procedure done by a doctor that is out of network, it may cost $20,000. The patient is then responsible for the deductible, which may be $2,000, and TRICARE may cover only 50 percent of the remainder amount of the procedure, or $9,000.
- Beneficiaries may see any TRICARE authorized provider they choose.
- The government will share the cost with the beneficiaries after deductibles.

TRICARE Extra is a preferred provider option (PPO) where you will choose a doctor, hospital, or other medical provider within the TRICARE provider network. You can locate a network provider by calling the local TRICARE service center or by visiting www.tricare.osd.mil/beneficiary/beneficiary/BCACdir/BCACview.aspx.

TRICARE Standard is a fee-for-service option. You can see an authorized TRICARE provider of your choice. Having this flexibility means that your care will usually cost more. For more information about fee-for-service, see Chapter 7.

TRICARE for Life

A military beneficiary who reaches age 65 and is eligible for Medicare Part A will become part of TRICARE for Life (TFL). TFL acts as a second payer; thus, after you go to the doctor and a bill is submitted for reimbursement, the bill iss submitted to Medicare first. Whatever is not covered by Medicare is submitted to TFL. Here are some of the perks of TRICARE for Life:
- There are no enrollment fees.
- You pay only the Medicare Part B premium.

• TRICARE pays for TRICARE benefits not covered by Medicare, such as pharmaceutical drugs.

TRICARE Plus

TRICARE Plus is a military treatment facility primary care enrollment program. It provides medical and/or dental care to eligible people at selective local military treatment facilities. All beneficiaries eligible for care in military treatment facilities (except those enrolled in TRICARE Prime, a civilian HMO, or Medicare HMO) can seek enrollment for primary care at military treatment facilities where enrollment capacity exists.

Many of the benefits and eligibility requirements vary depending on the location of the military treatment facilities. Local commanders will retain discretion to continue or discontinue TRICARE Plus at individual military treatment facilities depending on their capacities/capabilities and missions.

Some of the benefits include:

- A designated primary care provider at the military treatment facility is the principal source of healthcare.
- Those enrolled in TRICARE Plus can continue to obtain care from civilian and/or Medicare providers.
- TRICARE Standard/Extra or Medicare rules apply.
- TRICARE will be the second payer to Medicare for TRICARE-covered services.
- You are not locked into a health maintenance organization (HMO)-like program.
- There are no enrollment fees.
- Enrollees receive primary care appointments with the same access standards as TRICARE Prime enrollees have.
- Eenrollment is noted on beneficiary records in the Defense Enrollment Eligibility Reporting System (DEERS).
- If you have an existing relationship with certain primary care providers at military treatment facilities, you will have the first opportunity to enroll as long as the facility has the capacity (space) and capability (resources).

For more information, go to the TRICARE website at www.tricare.osd.mil/Plus or call the TRICARE information center at 888-DoD-LIFE (888-363-5433).

TRICARE Reserve Select (TRS)

Although TRS has some things in common with the other TRICARE programs, it cannot be directly compared to any of them. TRS is a premium-based insurance plan in which members enroll and must pay an enrollment premium. However, if payment is not made on time, you will be removed from the plan and may not enroll again later.

You do not use military treatment facilities or pharmacies. All of your doctor visits, hospitalizations, pharmacy, and ancillary care (i.e. lab work, x-rays, etc.) are given in the civilian network through a TRICARE-authorized provider. Under TRS, there are two types of coverage with separate premiums:

- TRS member-only coverage
- TRS member and family coverage

Due to the fact that this plan is so new, the information is vague.

To find out more information, go to www.tricare.osd.mil or call 877-874-2273.

Continued Health Care Benefit Program (CHCBP)

The Continued Health Care Benefit Program (CHCBP) provides military health benefits for former military beneficiaries who lost their military healthcare coverage or will lose it soon. It provides healthcare coverage to:

- Service members, who may also enroll their family members
- Certain former spouses of military members who have not remarried who was married for over 20 years (benefits can be further defined by a regional contractor at www.tricare.osd.mil)
- Children who have lost their military coverage due to age or marriage

CHCBP is a temporary insuranc plan that limits coverage to either 18 or 36 months. While it is not TRICARE, its benefits are comparable to the TRICARE Standard benefits, and covers preexisting conditions that may not be covered by a new employer's benefit plan. CHCBP follows most of the rules and procedures of TRICARE Standard. However, for some types of treatment, coverage can be limited. To determine what types of treatment have limited coverage, call the CHCBP administration at 800-444-5445 or go to the "TRICARE Handbook" at www.tricare.osd.mil/Tricare Handbook/.

You must enroll in CHCBP within 60 days of the loss of your rights in the military health system. To enroll, you will be required to submit:

- A completed CHCBP Enrollment Application form (DD Form 2837)
- Documentation as requested on the enrollment form (DD-214-Certificate of Release or Discharge from Active Duty; final divorce decree; DD1173-Uniformed Services ID Card; as well as additional information and documentation may be required to confirm an applicant's eligibility for CHCBP)
- A premium payment for the first 90 days of health coverage

The premium rates as of the publication of this book were $933 per quarter for individuals and $1,996 per quarter for families. These rates tend to change annually, so be sure to contact your Tricare/CHCBP representative to verify the current rates. CHCBP is run by Humana Military Healthcare Services, Inc., which will bill you for subsequent quarterly premiums until you are no longer eligible once your enrollment has begun. To find out more information, call 800-444-5445 or go online to www.humana-military.com.

Extended Care Health Option (ECHO) Program

On September 1, 2005, TRICARE's Extended Care Health Option (ECHO) replaced the TRICARE Program for Persons with Disabilities (PFPWD). Beneficiaries who still have authorization approvals for PFPWD can continue on those approvals until the expiration or services are requested and authorized under the ECHO program. To find out if you are eligible for the new program, go to www.tricare.osd.mil/echo/echo-eligibility.cfm.

This program provides financial assistance to active duty family members who have qualifying conditions such as: moderate or severe mental retardation, a serious physical disability, or an extraordinary physical or psychological condition of such complexity that they are required to stay at home.

ECHO increases the PFPWD's cost-share limit from $1,000 per month to $2,500 per month per eligible family member. In addition to other TRI-CARE ECHO benefits, if you are homebound, you may qualify for extended in-home healthcare services. Unfortunately, for this there is a benefit cap.

ECHO will require you to first use public funds and facilities if they are available and adequate for your needs, but only for a smaller subset of the ECHO benefits.

Under ECHO, you will be required to pay part of the monthly-authorized expenses for your family members, based on your pay grade. (For details, see the list on www.tricare.osd.mil/echo/faqs.cfm.)

ECHO offers an integrated set of services and supplies that will supplement the basic TRICARE program options: TRICARE Prime (including TRICARE Prime Remote for Active Duty Family Members), TRICARE Standard, or TRICARE Extra. For more information about the program, go to www.tricare.osd.mil/echo/default.cfm or contact or contact your regional contractor; you can find a list at www.tricare.osd.mil/echo/echo-resources.cfm.

Veterans Administration Benefits

The most popular health coverage for past and present members of the armed forces is the Department of Veterans Affairs (VA) health system. As of 2005, there were about 163 VA hospitals around the country. To be eligible for VA assistance:

- You must be of veteran status. This means you had active duty service in the military, naval, or air service, and also had a discharge or release from that service under anything other than dishonorable conditions.
- Some veterans must have completed 24 continuous months of active military service. There are some exceptions to this, including: returning service members such as reservists and national guard called to active duty, those who served in other capacities aside from combat, those discharged for reasons other than dishonorable condition, women, and others. A more extensive list may be found at www.va.gov/healtheligibility/home/othergroups.asp or by calling 877-222-VETS.

• You must be recently discharged from the military for a disability determined to have been incurred or been aggravated in the line of duty.

There are a number of groups that have provided military-related service to the United States and, because of this, have been granted VA benefits. For this service to qualify, the secretary of defense must certify that your group has provided active military service. Individuals must be issued a discharge by the secretary of defense to qualify for VA benefits. To find out if you qualify, contact the Department of Veterans Affairs at 877-222-VETS (877-222-8387) or go to www.va.gov/healtheligibility/home/othergroups.asp#us.

You may enroll online at https://www.1010ez.med.va.gov/sec/vha/1010ez/. Once you apply for enrollment, your eligibility will be verified. The number of veterans who can be enrolled in the healthcare program is determined by the amount of money Congress gives the VA each year. Since funds are limited, the VA sets up priority groups to make sure that certain groups of veterans are able to be enrolled before others. Based on your specific eligibility status, you will be assigned a priority group ranging from 1 to 8, 1 being the highest priority for enrollment. Some veterans may have to agree to pay copay to be placed in certain priority groups.

In addition, you may be eligible for more than one enrollment priority group. In that case, the VA will always place you in the highest priority group that you are eligible for. Under the Medical Benefits Package, the same services are generally available to all enrolled veterans. The priority groups are complicated and some reference financial thresholds. For more information about the thresholds, go to the "Copays and Charges" page at www.va.gov/healtheligibility/costs/costs.asp or www.va.gov/health eligibility/eligibility/epg_all.asp to find out your priority eligibility.

In general, benefits may include:
• Basic care
• Preventive care
• Periodic medical exams
• Health education, including nutrition education
• Maintenance of drug use profiles, drug monitoring, and drug use education
• Mental health and substance abuse preventive services

- Outpatient medical, surgical and mental healthcare, including care for substance abuse
- Inpatient hospital, medical, surgical, and mental healthcare, including care for substance abuse
- Prescription drugs, including over-the-counter drugs and medical and surgical supplies available under the VA's own system of determining prices
- Emergency care in VA facilities
- Durable medical equipment and prosthetic and orthotic devices, including eyeglasses and hearing aids
- Home health services
- Respite, hospice, and palliative care
- Pregnancy and delivery service to the extent authorized by law (if a procedure is illegal, the VA will not perform it)

There are several new and obscure programs offered to those VA beneficiaries. One such program is offered to Vietnam veterans with type 2 diabetes might be eligible for disability compensation from the Department of Veterans Affairs (VA) based on their presumed exposure to Agent Orange or other herbicides.

The evidence of a link between exposure to Agent Orange, dioxin, the problematic contaminant in Agent Orange, and diabetes is modest. Most of the association between Agent Orange and diabetes comes from studies of people who lived near or worked at manufacturing plants that produced large quantities of Agent Orange toxin. In those cases, there seems to be some relationship between Agent Orange exposure and increased insulin resistance, the precursor to type 2 diabetes. Other conditions that are included on this list are:

- Adult-onset (Type 2) diabetes
- Chronic lymphocytic leukemia (CLL)
- Hodgkin's disease
- Multiple myeloma
- Non-Hodgkin's lymphoma
- Acute and subacute peripheral neuropathy
- Porphyria cutanea tarda, chloracne, prostate cancer
- Respiratory cancers (cancer of the lung, bronchus, larynx, or trachea)

• Soft-tissue sarcoma (other than osteosarcoma, chondrosarcoma, Kaposi's sarcoma, or mesothelioma)

In general, the exposure that Vietnam veterans had to Agent Orange was much less than the populations studied by scientists. Still, the VA has added diabetes to the list of conditions for which Vietnam veterans are eligible for disability compensation. Vietnam veterans who are interested in participating in this Agent Orange program should contact the nearest VA medical center for an examination. If it is ruled that the diabetes is an onset of Agent Orange and service related, the VA would pay disability compensation. To find out more about Agent Orange, go to www1.va.gov/agentorange /docs/AOIB10-49JUL03.pdf. To find out more information on VA benefits and special programs that may be offered through the VA, go to www.va.gov/healtheligibility/home/hecmain.asp.

Other healthcare programs include the Children of Vietnam Veterans, such as those born with birth defects like spina bifida. The VA provides certain benefits for children with birth defects who were born to female Vietnam veterans. These programs are administered by the Health Administration Center. For more information about these programs, go to www.va.gov/hac.

The VA also provides a onetime payment of no more than $11,000 toward the purchase of an automobile or other vehicle, including adaptive equipment and for repair, replacement, or reinstallation required because of disability under disability insurance. To qualify, you must have either:

• A service-connected loss or permanent loss of use of one or both hands or feet; or
• A permanent impairment of vision of both eyes to a certain degree; or
• Entitlement to compensation for ankylosis (immobility) of one or both knees or one or both hips

To apply for this benefit or request further information, contact your nearest VA health benefits and service center at www1.va.gov/health_ benefits/ or calling 800-827-1000.

There are several other healthcare-related programs for VA beneficiaries, from travel reimbursement for medical visits to assistance for home improvement where medically necessary to specially equipped computers for the blind. By doing the research and asking questions until you get acceptable answers or feel comfortable with the answers you are given as well as being persistant and if the person does not anwer your question to what you deem acceptible, ask to speak to their supervisor or to someone who might be able to answer your question completely. In the end, you may be surprised to find that most of your medical benefits are covered.

Civilian Health and Medical Program of the Uniformed Services (CHAMPUS)

This program, now called TRICARE, is explained in detail above. Retirees, spouses, and children of active-duty, retired, and deceased members of the armed forces can be covered by an insurance company called the Civilian Health and Medical Program of the Uniformed Services. This program will pay for the use of nonmilitary medical services

CHAMPUS is a federally funded health program that provides beneficiaries with medical care supplemental to that available in military and Public Health Service (PHS) facilities. All CHAMPUS beneficiaries move over to Medicare at age 65. CHAMPUS is like Medicare in that the government contracts with private parties to administer the program.

CHAPTER 11

FSAs, HSAs, and HRAs

O NE OF THE NEWER TRENDS IN healthcare are healthcare accounts that can be used to help fund employee healthcare
expenses. They are: flexible spending accounts (FSAs), health savings accounts (HSAs), and health reimbursement arrangements (HRAs). If
you are in a higher tax bracket and are looking for an investment vehicle, or
who need tax benefits, you might want to investigate one of the following
options further.

Flexible Spending Account (FSA)

Your employer may offer a flexible spending plan, also called a cafeteria
plan, which allows you to put your pretax dollars into an account under
Section 125 of the Internal Revenue Code. According to this plan, you are
reimbursed for your out-of-pocket medical expenses, such as prescription
drugs, dental care, and copayments, as they occur.

Because flexible spending contributions are taken out of your pay before
federal and state taxes are calculated, it's your pretax dollars that pay your
medical bills. If you know you have certain fixed medical expenses every
year (such as pharmaceutical or psychiatric expenses) that are not covered
by your health insurance plan, you should definitely take advantage of your
flexible spending account. The more pretax dollars used (tax exempt) to pay
for medical expenses, the better off you will be.

How Does an FSA Work?

The employee contributes an amount of their choosing to this account through a salary reduction agreement. You are then able to withdraw the funds from your paycheck via your FSA to pay for any medical bills.

The salary reduction agreement means that the funds you set aside are put into a flexible spending account and escape both income tax and Social Security tax. Employers may contribute to these accounts as well. There is no statutory limit on the amount of money that can be contributed to flexible spending accounts. However, some companies place a limit of $2,000 to $3,000 on flexible spending accounts.

Under IRS regulations, the amount of the reduction cannot be changed and the employee cannot drop out of the plan within the fiscal year. However, there is a loophole that allows you to change your status if you have experienced a large change in your family status (e.g. birth, adoption, marriage, divorce, loss of a dependent, or termination of a spouse's employment).

By law, you forfeit any unspent funds in your account at the end of the year. However, a new provision was enacted for the 2005 tax year that extends this rule two and a half months. This means you will have an extra two and a half months to use these funds after December 31. This provision is explained in the IRS's Publication 553.

Your employer must make available to you the full amount of the benefit whenever reimbursable expenses occur. for example, an employee who designates $1,800 per year (equal to a payroll deduction of $150 per month) is eligible for reimbursement of up to $1,800 in the first month of the plan year if there are expenses of that amount—even though only $150 has been paid into the account at that time.

When you use a FSA, you can reduce your taxable income and use that income reduction to pay for expenses that normally would have been paid with after-tax dollars. These tax savings include federal income tax, and in most jurisdictions, state and local income taxes. In addition, employees do not pay Social Security and Medicare tax (7.65 percent) on the amount excluded from your income.

Is an FSA Right for Me?

There are some side effects. When your salary is reduced, your employer's costs for benefits related to your salary may also decrease. Other salary-related benefits that may result in employer savings other than Medicare and

Social Security include the following: unemployment and worker's compensation, short- and long-term disability coverage, life insurance, and pension. Unless the pension statutes or ordinances are revised, your employer's funding and your pension benefits in many plans will be based on the reduced salary.

Unfortunately, if a benefit is based on salary, the benefit will be reduced unless plans are revised to avoid those reductions. Your pension will probably be the first benefit for you to review. If you are close to termination or retirement, you will be impacted most severely because those pension benefits are often based on your average salary for the last several years of employment. FSA may not be the best option for you.

Life insurance and disability benefits are also typically based on your salary. Your employer has discretion to determine whether the full or reduced salary is used to compute these benefits. Because FSAs are advantageous to employers, they are usually willing to base these benefit amounts on the full salary to encourage participation, but you should check to make sure what happens in your specific office.

Workers compensation and unemployment benefits are based on the average monthly wage. For those who earn above the maximum monthly wage, benefits would not be reduced. However, for lower income employees, the reduction in potential benefits could be substantial. This differs from state to state, as state law dictates whether or not these benefits can be based on full salary. To find out more information on your maximum monthly wage, your potential reduction in benefits, etc., call your state department of labor. You can locate your state department of labor at http://workforce security.doleta.gov/map.asp.

Social Security benefits are based on salary throughout an employee's career, so your retirement benefits should not be significantly reduced, particularly if the FSA reduction does not occur over your entire career. However, if you are new to the workplace and have selected a large reduction, this could cause you to receive a significantly lower Social Security disability benefit if you become disabled.

Likewise, the survivor benefits could also be significantly lower. Survivor benefits are those that benefit from a deceased person's benefits such as the wife of a deceased husband. for example, if the husband worked at his job for a "short amount of time" before he or she was injured or retired, and suddenly died, the wife of that person (or person he or she supported) would receive his or her benefits. Since the amount of time and salary dictate most your monetary social security benefits, working less time at a lower salary will leave you with less money in your social security, thus resulting is "less benefits" for you and your spouse. Benefits may vary from state to state, so it is best to contact your state social security office to clarify any benefits or new regulations. Your state social security administration can be located at www.ncsssa.org/ssaframes.html.

Health Savings Accounts (HSAs); Medical Savings Accounts

This is another alternative to healthcare insurance that may be more beneficial. A health savings account (HSA), otherwise known as a medical savings account, allows you, your family members, and your employers to make tax-deductible cash contributions to a frozen account.

In other words, it is an individual health spending account that is owned by you and may be used for payments of current and future unreimbursed medical expenses, or as retirement income. You can use these funds to reimburse you (tax-free) for qualifying medical expenses. They are meant exclusively to pay qualified medical expenses of the beneficiary of the account.

A medical savings account is not an insurance plan. It's actually a means of making coverage more affordable for people who traditionally have high health insurance costs. Here's how the health savings plan works: rather than pay a high monthly premium for a policy with a low deductible and low copays, you opt for a high deductible policy (to help in the event of an emergency or major expense) *and* you make regular deposits into a healthcare savings account (to cover the minor expenses).

For example, an individual can contribute and deduct up to $2,600 in contributions per year. However, there is no need to put the maximum amount of money into the account to set it up. (The limit is twice as high for families.)

The money you put into the HSA is tax-deductible and your account grows tax-free, similar to an individual retirement account (IRA). You can make tax-free withdrawals to pay for any IRS-approved medical expenses, as defined in the IRS Code, Section 213(d) at http://specialneedschildren.com/about/irc213.html, and there is no need for HMO approvals. IRS 2005 Publication 502 at www.irs.gov/pub/irs-pdf/p502.pdf contains a list of medical expenses you can use for deductions that you can submit for payment from your flexible spending account; however, this is not a comprehensive list. These expenses include, but are not limited to, medical plan deductibles, diagnostic services covered by your plan, long-term care insurance premiums, and health insurance premiums if you are receiving federal unemployment compensation, over-the-counter drugs, LASIK surgery, and some nursing services. Also keep in mind that only some insurance premiums are considered "qualified medical expenses." Be clarify definitions and conditions, sure to contact the IRS at 800-829-3676 or your accountant to verify this list or find out if there were any recent changes to this list. In addition, whatever you don't spend it this year, rolls over to future years for medical expenses and keeps growing—tax-free. Deposits made towards your health savings plan are 100 percent tax-deductible and can be used toward any of your out-of-pocket medical expenses (satisfying your deductible, covering office visits, etc). Any health savings account funds you don't use will remain in the account, drawing interest on a tax-favored basis, until needed for future medical expenses or retirement.

In order to qualify, you must be covered by a high-deductible health insurance plan and be either self-employed or employed by a firm with 50 or fewer employees. Any individual covered under a qualified "high deductible" health plan (and not covered by certain other health plans, such as that of a spouse's employer) may also establish an HSA. Many of the enrollment requirements can be found in the IRS publication 969 and the instructions in form number 8889. Go to www.irs.gov/pub/irs-pdf/p969.pdf for the full description of the document.

HSA's High Deductible Health Plan Option
Included in the HSA is a High Deductible Health Plan (HDHP) option. This health plan has deductibles of at least $1,000 for individual coverage and $2,000 for family coverage. Typically, the deductibles in these plans are considerably higher than the minimum levels of the typical HSA, thus the name "High Deductible Health Plan option." Total out-of-pocket expenses (deductibles, copayments, etc.) cannot exceed $5,000 for an individual and $10,000 per family. You are responsible for all healthcare after this limit is reached. The deductible and out-of-pocket limits are reviewed yearly and checked if they need to change due to.

HDHPs may, but are not required to, provide first-dollar coverage, with no deductible, for specified preventive care services. In its simplest terms, this means that instead of buying a health insurance policy with a $250 deductible, you would buy a policy with a $2,500 deductible. It costs a lot less every month, but you must pay for the first $2,500 in medical expenses each year. The deductible applies to all services and medical expenses, including most prescription drug expenses, except for those expenses from preventive care.

How Do HSA Plans Compare to Traditional Plans?

When you compare a traditional HMO plan to an HSA plan, you'll notice that the two are comparable. For example, your traditional health policy has a $250 annual deductible, and no copayments above that amount. Your premium for this plan would be roughly $300 a month, or $3,600 a year. Under HSA's high-deductible plan, your deductible is $2,500 and there are no copayments above that amount. Your annual premium is about $1,560. You could also deduct the monthly cost of this premium from your taxes, but certain circumstances may apply.

The apparent saving between the two plans is about $2,000 per year. If the $1,560 premium is made tax-deductible, that will increase. For example, individuals in the 35 percent tax bracket would have an after-tax premium cost of only about $950 per year. While it may appear that you saved money, you will actually be depositing that amount into your tax-deductible HSA account. You will then be able to withdraw this money tax-free to pay your first $2,500 of medical expenses, if they occur.

As you can see, if you do not have the money to pay the $3,600 annual premium for traditional healthcare, you can purchase high-deductible insurance and place a small amount into your HSA account. Nothing says you have to deposit the entire $2,000 or $2,500 savings in the HSA. But later in the year, if you do have medical expenses, make sure you put the money in so you get the tax deduction *first,* and *then* pay the bills from that account.

Who Can Enroll and How to Fund Your HSA

If you are younger than 65, not covered by other health insurance (except for insurance that provides preventive care or specific disease coverage), and cannot be claimed as a dependent on someone else's tax return, you are eligible to enroll in an HSA account. Something to keep in mind, however: if you are 65 or older, you cannot open or join an employer-sponsored HSAs, but you may continue to use funds from your already existing HSA.

HDHP deductible totals in 2005 were $1,000 for a minimum annual deductible and a maximum annual deductible and other out-of-pocket expenses of $5,100 for individuals and $2,000 minimum annual deductible and a maximum annual deductible and other out-of-pocket expenses of $10,200 for families. These limits do not apply to deductibles and expenses for out-of-network services if the plan uses a network of providers. Instead, only deductibles and out-of-pocket expenses for services within the network should be used to figure whether the limit applies. The maximum you or your employers can contribute to your medical savings account is 65 percent of the deductible (for single coverage) of your health plan and 75 percent of the deductible (for family coverage) of your health plan. For example, if you have a health plan with a deductible of $2,225, then you can contribute up to $1,446.25 to your medical savings account. If you are on the family plan with a deductible of $4,500, your maximum contribution is $3,375. Employers must make comparable contributions on behalf of all participating employees. Basically, contributions must be the same dollar amount or the same percentage of the employees deductible for all employees in the same class. What is meant by class is either "individual" versus "family" and "self-only coverage" versus "family coverage." Also keep in mind that if your employee makes contributions to your HSA that the contribution is *not* tax-deductible to you, the employee (it is excluded from your income).

HSAs must be funded through a trust or custodial account similar to a deferred compensation or 401(k) account. First of all, a trust is a legal entity in which assets are actually owned and held on behalf of the beneficiary, thus the trustee must exercise discretionary authority in the best interests of the beneficiary. On the other hand, in a custodial account, the "custodian" holds the assets on behalf of the owner of the assets. However, both may have slightly different definitions depending on the state in which you live. A model Health Savings Trust account agreement form 5305-B (approved by the IRS) may be found at www.irs.gov/pub/irs-pdf/f5305b.pdf, and a model of a custodial HSA account agreement (approved by the IRS) may be found at: www.irs.gov/pub/irs-pdf/f5305c.pdf. Be sure to check with www.irs.gov for possible updates of these forms.

With all the above said, the only way to establish one of these accounts is through an approved institution. These approved institutions include insured banks and credit unions or any other entity that currently meets the IRS standards for being a trustee or custodian for an IRA or Archer Medical Savings Account (MSA) may be an HSA trustee or custodian. The law also allows insurance companies to be HSA trustees or custodians. If you are unsure if your bank, credit union, or insurance company is qualified to offer an HSA, or you are unsure where to start, check websites such as www.hsainsider.com for companies that will be willing to establish your account regardless of where you live.

Funds from your HSA can be used, pretax, to pay for qualified medical expenses (medical care, prescription, and nonprescription medications), and long-term care insurance premiums as a result of unemployment, COBRA (see Chapter 12 for more information) and Medicare Part B (see Chapter 8 for more information).

HSA funds are owned completely by the account holder. For an HSA established by an employee, the employee, the employee's employer or both may contribute to the HSA of the employee in a given year. For an HSA established by a self-employed (or unemployed) individual, the individual may contribute to the HSA. Family members may also make contributions to an HSA on behalf of another family member as long as that other family member is an eligible individual (i.e., a trustee or custodian as described above).

The contribution limit for an individual who begins self-only coverage under an HDHP is computed each month. For example, if the annual deductible is $5,000 for the HDHP, the lesser of the annual deductible and $2,600 is $2,600. The monthly contribution limit is $216.67 ($2,600/12). The annual contribution limit is $1,516.69 (7 x $216.67).

In addition, HSA funds may be carried over from year to year, regardless of your employment status and are portable from employer to employer, much like an IRA. These funds are not taxable, either as the account grows or when it is used to pay for eligible medical expenses, unless funds are withdrawn for nonmedical purposes. Funds used for nonmedical purposes will be taxed and penalized in a similar manner to those from an IRA (they are subject to income tax plus a 10 percent penalty and additional tax). This penalty does not apply after death, disability, or after an individual attains Medicare eligibility (age 65). At this point the account is simply subject to an ordinary income tax and not a penalty tax. In the event of death, the surviving spouse is subject to income tax only if distributions from the HSA are not used for qualified medical expenses.

To see a more thorough breakdown of this plan, go to www.healthplanspecialists.com and click on the HSA audio and visual presentation. Different states may have variations on the requirements, so be sure to check with your state insurance department at www.healthinsurance finders.com/cr_state_department_ of_insurance.html.

Health Reimbursement Accounts or Arrangements (HRAs)

HRAs are conceptually similar to HSAs but are completely controlled by the employer. HRAs are also used to pay for qualified medical expenses, but may be also used to reimburse employees for the purchase of traditional health insurance. There is no requirement that these accounts be prefunded, vested or linked to a HDHP. Typically, the employer does not specifically set money aside to cover employees, instead, he or she reimburses you for eligible medical expenses from the general operating funds. Although it is not required, HRAs are usually accompanied by a high deductible health plan. Some of these "eligible medical expenses" include the following:

- Acupuncture
- Ambulance service
- Birth control pills
- Chiropractic care
- Contact lenses (corrective)★
- Dental fees★
- Diagnostic tests
- Doctors' fees
- Drug addiction/alcoholism treatment
- Drugs (prescription and some over-the-counter nonprescription only)★
- Experimental medical treatment
- Eyeglasses (corrective)★
- Guide dogs
- Hearing aids and exams
- Injections and vaccinations

- In vitro fertilization
- Nursing services★
- Optometrist fees
- Orthodontic treatment★
- Prescription drugs to alleviate nicotine withdrawal symptoms
- Smoking cessation programs/treatments
- Surgery★
- Transportation for local medical care
- Wheelchairs
- X-rays
- Under the CommonHealth program, fees for health and bone density screenings and flu shots

★Limited reimbursement

For a more comprehensive list, visit www.irs.gov and go to Publication 502, located at www.irs.gov/pub/irs-pdf/p502.pdf.

An HRA is available only through an employer and must be funded solely by the employer. The employer owns the account—unlike an HSA, which is owned by you, the individual. Because of this, the employer has the authority to decide to carry over money from one year to the next. Even if the employer does elect to allow carryovers, it may cap the carryover amount. Employers also have the power to decide whether to give former employees access to their accrued HRA money, and what it is used for.

Generally, all unused funds are rolled over at the end of the year. Former employees, including retirees, have continued access to unused reimbursement money. HRAs remain with the original employer and do not follow you to new employment. Because of this, an HSA is a better option than an HRA; however, this account may still be a better option than a healthy individual paying high monthly premiums and getting nothing in return.

One of the reasons employers like HRAs is that it qualifies them for preferential tax treatment of those funds. Employers can deduct the cost of an insurance plan—and health reimbursement accounts—as a business expense under Internal Revenue Code Section 162.

Both the HSA and HRA spending accounts should provide first dollar coverage; i.e., the dollar amount should be matched one to one for specified preventive care. Keep in mind that certain prescription drugs, such as those used to prevent a heart attack, treat obesity, or help quit smoking, also count as preventive care and are covered. When negotiating for healthcare, be sure to specify that the plan provides coverage of allowable preventive care, without your needing to pay the deductible first.

CHAPTER 12

COBRA

THANKS TO THE CONSOLIDATED Omnibus Budget Rec-onciliation Act (COBRA) of 1986, you can now change jobs without worrying about a lapse in your health insurance. COBRA insurance allows you to keep your health insurance for you and your family through certain events: death of a covered employee, unemployment, divorce, a child's loss of dependent status, or becoming entitled to Medicare.

What this means is that you are guaranteed by federal law the right to continue your former employer's group plan as an individual or family healthcare coverage for up to 18 months at your own expense. Your spouse and dependent children are also eligible for COBRA coverage, sometimes for as long as three years. However, any plans you may have purchased inde-pendently of your employer are not subject to COBRA law.

Who Is Eligible for COBRA Coverage?

There are three groups of people who are eligible for COBRA coverage: employees or former employees in a private business with at least 20 employees, their spouses, and their dependent children. One of several types of "qualifying events" must occur in order to trigger COBRA, such as:
- Job termination
- Reduced hours
- Employee entitled to Medicare
- Divorce or legal separation
- Death of employee
- Loss of dependent-child status
- Bankruptcy of employer

You are eligible to buy COBRA for the maximum coverage period as determined by your status and which event occurred. Your COBRA coverage can last from 18 months (for losing your job) to 36 months (for a divorcee). At any time during this period, you can choose to obtain another type of healthcare coverage.

COBRA eligibility is extended to workers in state and local government, as well as to independent contractors. This law excludes the District of Columbia, all federal employees, certain church-related organizations, and firms employing fewer than 20 people (however employers must include their part-time workers to determine if they are exempt).

If you work at a small company that is exempt from federal law, you are not completely out of luck. Many states have adopted their own laws, sometimes known as "mini-COBRA," that often grant broader rights to determine your eligibility for coverage. Check with your state insurance department (you can locate most of the state's websites at www.naic.org/state_web_map.htm) to find out if you are entitled to continued healthcare coverage under a state COBRA plan.

If you are applying for COBRA under job termination, this includes voluntarily resignation from a job or termination—for any reason except "gross misconduct."

If you elect COBRA continuation coverage when you are working, i.e. when you decide to accept your former job's healthcare plan instead of your new employment, you can keep your health coverage but you must pay the full premium. In some states, Medicaid helps pay for the premium. Contact the Department of Labor (DOL) at 1-866-444-3272, or access DOL's website at www.dol.gov.

Employers with self-funded health plans (generally large corporations) are exempt from state regulation of their plans, but employers that buy coverage through outside insurers (generally smaller businesses) are subject to their state's laws.

In addition, you must also be covered under your employer's health plan originally to be eligible for COBRA. If your employer has more than 20 workers, but doesn't offer health coverage, or offers coverage to only certain groups of employees and you're not one of them, you won't be eligible for COBRA, even if one of the "qualifying events" occurs—nor will your spouse or children be eligible.

Costs and Length of Coverage

Your COBRA coverage ends when:

- You reach the last day of maximum coverage
- Premiums are not paid on a timely basis
- The employer ceases to maintain any group health plan
- You obtain coverage through another employer group health plan that does not contain any exclusion or limitation with respect to any pre-existing condition of a beneficiary
- A beneficiary is entitled to Medicare benefits

The cost of your monthly premiums once you begin COBRA coverage can come as quite a surprise if you're accustomed to your employer picking up most of your health insurance tab via pre-paycheck deductions. When you opt to buy COBRA, you must pay the full premium amount, plus administrative fees of at least 2 percent.

To get a better idea for how much this may cost, call the HR department of your company and ask for the amount your employer is paying for a person's full premium coverage. For example, if your coverage cost $600 a month, you might have been paying only $60 a month while your employer was paying the rest. To this total, you will add a 2 percent administration fee. This will be the most you would expect to pay if you select to keep your benefits. In this example, you would keep all your benefits through COBRA for a monthly cost of $612 for 18 months.

Disabled beneficiaries can expect to receive an additional 11 months of coverage after the initial 18 months. However, the premium for those extra months may be increased to 150 percent of the plan's total cost of coverage; this is determined by your employer.

If your medical and dental expenses exceed 7.5 percent of your adjusted gross income, you can take a tax deduction on that amount. For more information on the Health Coverage Tax Credit, call 1-866-628-2282 or visit the website at www.irs.gov by entering the keyword "HCTC."

Why COBRA Coverage Could Work for You

COBRA may be a good option for people who have preexisting conditions, as it allows you to continue your already existing coverage while you look for other options. It's important to have coverage because almost all insurers will consider your health when deciding whether or not to offer you insurance. Insurance companies can reject you for coverage completely—or exclude coverage of your existing condition. Some states, like Washington, ban this practice. Federal law forbids all group health plans, such as Kaiser, Blue Cross Blue Shield etc from medically underwriting you i.e. screening prospective health care plan members out of the plan on the basis of health or pre-existing medical condition which is currently not legal in Washington. Remember, COBRA is a continuation of existing coverage, so you will not have to deal with "underwriting" which categorizes a patient into a certain health plan based on his/her previous medical history.

The federal Health Insurance Portability and Accountability Act (HIPAA) guarantees that people who have continuous health coverage— cannot be denied insurance even if they have preexisting conditions. Because of this, if you decide not to take COBRA and create a gap in your coverage, you would lose your HIPAA protection when you decide to buy insurance later in your life.

You should also consider the extent of your health plan benefits and your network of doctors and other healthcare providers. If you have the choice between your spouse's healthcare plan and continuing COBRA coverage, if your old plan has extensive benefits, you might want to stay with it. Always check if you will lose your doctors if you switch your plan.

Your COBRA coverage must remain identical to the coverage you had before. Employers can—but are not required to—give you the option of dropping such non-core benefits as dental and vision care. If you were covered by, for example, three different health plans at the same time (one for hospitalization, another for prescriptions, and a third for medical), you have the right to continue coverage in any or all of them.

If you decide to continue coverage with COBRA, you should choose to continue the exact same coverage. If you do not, it may appear to a third party insurer that a new health problem has developed. This would make it more difficult to obtain other health insurance coverage after your COBRA period expires.

Continuing COBRA Coverage

In order to continue healthcare coverage with COBRA, you must follow certain guidelines in order to avoid a potential drop in coverage.

- Both you and your employer must follow proper procedure to initiate COBRA, or else you could forfeit your rights to coverage.
- The employer must notify the health plan administrator (typically, the employer; or the person in which you mail your premium payments to) within 30 days after an employee's death, job termination, reduced hours of employment, or eligibility for Medicare.
- In cases of divorce, legal marital separation, or a child's loss of dependent status, it is your (or your family's) responsibility to notify the health plan administrator within 60 days.
- The plan administrator has 14 days to alert you and your family members—in person or by first-class mail—about your rights to COBRA. If the plan administrator fails to act, he or she can be held personally liable by the IRS for a breach of duties.

There are two exceptions to the notification rule, if the plan allows them. The first is the time limit for both notification periods can be extended. The second, is that the employer may be relieved of their obligation to notify the plan administrators that the employees quit or reduced their work hours. It is then up to the plan administrator to determine if a qualifying event has occurred. You should find out in advance what your health plan allows.

You, your spouse, and your children have 60 days to decide whether to buy COBRA. The 60 days begins from the day your eligibility notification is sent to you or the day that you lost your health coverage—whichever is later. Your coverage will work retroactively to the date that you lost your benefits (as long as you pay the premium).

During this 60 day period, you might initially decide not to take COBRA coverage and waive your rights. However, as long as those 60 days have not ended, at any time you can change your mind and revoke your waiver. Your COBRA coverage would start the day your waiver was revoked. In this case, if you visited a doctor during the period you initially waived your COBRA rights, you will not be reimbursed for that claim, even if you later decide to buy COBRA. Below are a few other things you should keep in mind:

- **Premium payments.** After you select COBRA, you must pay your first premium within 45 days. This first premium is likely to be high because it covers the period retroactive to the date coverage ended through your employer. Your premiums should be paid every month according to health plan requirements, but COBRA rules allow for a 30-day grace period for each payment.

- **Extensions.** Although COBRA sets specific time limits on coverage, there is nothing stopping the health plan from extending your benefits beyond the coverage period. The key here is to ask your health provider.

- **Notification rights.** The U.S. Department of Labor (DOL) has jurisdiction over issues involving notification of private-sector employees about COBRA coverage. Employers that fail to comply with the notification rules face fines of up to $110 for every day that no notice is sent after the deadline. In addition, the IRS can assess an excise tax against any company that does not comply with COBRA regulations.

- **Life insurance.** COBRA makes no provisions for life insurance.

- **New workers.** If you are a newly hired employee, you must be given an initial general notice about your COBRA rights. Because COBRA is a federal law, the U.S. Department of Labor (DOL) has jurisdiction over issues involving notification of about COBRA coverage. Employers that fail to comply with the notification rules face fines of up to $110 for every day that no notice is sent after the deadline. In addition, the IRS can assess an excise tax against any company that does not comply with COBRA regulations.

- **Plan description.** COBRA information must be included in the summary of the health plan description you receive when you are new to the plan.

- **Switching plans.** If your employer offers an open enrollment period to active employees and you are currently on COBRA coverage, you must be given the option to switch plans during that time.

- **Conversion plans.** If your health plan has the option to convert from a group plan to an individual policy under COBRA, you must be given that option and allowed to convert within 180 days before your COBRA coverage ends. At that point you will pay individual, not group, rates. Switching to individual coverage could weaken any HIPAA protections you have.

- **Moving.** If you relocate out of your COBRA health plan's coverage area, you will lose your COBRA benefits. Your old employer is
not required to offer you a plan in your new area.
- **Premium costs.** Your premiums can be increased if the costs of
the health plan increase for everyone at the workplace. Generally
they must be fixed in advance of each 12-month cycle. The plan
must allow you to pay your premiums on a monthly basis.
- **Premium notices.** No one (including your health plan and the
employer) is required to send you monthly premium bills. Make
sure you pay attention to your due dates.
- **Disability.** If you are eligible for Social Security disability benefits,
your COBRA coverage can last for no more than 29 months.
Employers can only cancel your COBRA coverage if they eliminate their group health coverage completely.

In addition, your COBRA coverage will be cancelled if you:
- Fail to make full and timely payments
- Become entitled to Medicare
- Obtain coverage under another group health plan after electing
COBRA
- Move out of the health plan's service area

For more information about COBRA, contact the Department of
Labor (DOL) at 1-866-444-3272, or access DOL's website at
www.dol.gov/ebsa if you were employed by a private sector employer. If
you were employed by a state or local government, you should contact the
nearest office of Wage and Hour Division. It's listed in most telephone
directories under Employee Standards Administration, U.S. Government, or
Department of Labor. You can also go to COBRA's website at
www.dol.gov/dol/topic/health-plans/cobra.htm or call 1-866-444-3272
(1-800-325-0778 for the speech impaired). A small booklet of COBRA
information can be requested from (202) 693-8664.

PART III

PITFALLS TO AVOID
AND
TIPS FOR SAVING

CHAPTER 13

WHAT IS PREVENTION?

A S SIMPLE AS IT SOUNDS, one of the most effective ways to lower your medical expenses over time is to prevent illness before it starts. By maintaining a healthy lifestyle and incorporating preventive health measures, you can take advantage of wellness programs provided by your health insurance and even kick unhealthy habits. Here are three things you can do to lower your medical expenses:

- Maintain a healthy weight
- Exercise regularly
- Have regular checkups

Today, more patients head for doctor's office for checkups than for any other reason. While you may assume that there is a blueprint all doctors follow, there's still lots of debate in the medical profession over which tests should be performed, on whom, beginning when and how often.

Unfortunately, there's not really a standard "one-size-fits-all" package. In order for your checkups to be really effective, they need to be tailored according to your age, sex, family history, and personal risk factors.

Some routine tests, such as electrocardiograms, chest x-rays, and full blood screening, actually provide little benefit if you are healthy. In fact, these health checkup schemes have only become so popular because they bring in the money! Running "routine" tests that will seldom catch a abnormality but that cost a lot is a very lucrative business. It's an additional bonus when a screening test picks up something dangerous, creating a patient who needs immediate attention.

It's good to mention here that there are definite perks to these screening tests. When they pick up on a disease in its early stages, it is much easier to treat and cure (for example, benign colon polyps, which become cancerous if not caught early).

The major drawback of the tests is that they are not very accurate. In other words, there are a large number of "false positives"; in other words, abnormal test results that require retesting (and thus create more stress and anxiety) but are not actually signs of an illness.

The only routine tests that the U.S. Preventive Services Task Force recommends are those for blood pressure, cholesterol, colorectal cancer, breast cancer, and cervical cancer. The task force refused to recommend screening against other diseases because either the current tests were not found to have merit, or there was not enough evidence to prove their benefit. As a bit of a catch-22, some tests actually could have a major negative impact on your health. They should be undertaken with a great deal of caution. For example, testing for cancer genes does nothing but tell you that you have the gene. It doesn't mean you will then have the disease, but knowing about the gene may cause you to become concerned or depressed over the possibility.

Here is a list of tests that should be viewed with caution if your doctor requests you to take them:

- **Chest x-ray.** This test is not recommended as part of your periodic medical examination unless you have signs, symptoms, or a change of status in a chronic condition. If your primary care physician feels you have some of the signs, symptoms, or change of status, ask what they are and be sure that a board certified radiologist is interpreting and performing the study because he or she is the only ones qualified to do this. Also, ask for a copy of the report to be sent home so you and your primary care doctor can review the results because a chest x-ray is interpreted by a radiologist, who is not your primary care doctor, but is a procedure that your primary care doctor requests you to have to better survey your condition and decide what treatments would be best for you.
- **Spirometry.** Unless you are suffering from significant shortness of breath, prolonged cough, or wheezing, your primary care physician should not recommend this test. If you do, you should have a board certified pumonologist perform the test. An internist may be able to handle the straightforward type of spirometry, but not the complex stage of the disease.

- **Blood tests.** If you do not have a family history of blood disease or cholesterol problems, you will rarely (if ever) need a complete workup. However, a fasting cholesterol test should be done every once in a while after the age of twenty. See the chart later in this chapter for specifics. Be wary if your physician has his own private lab in his office. His lab may not be covered by your insurance. In addition, it may be serviced by the receptionist or other part-time help rather than a full-time lab technician. Because of this inexperience, more false positives may occur—resulting in more money out of your pocket and incorrect readings. If the doctor sends the blood work out to an independent lab, check if your insurance will accept it.

- **Sigmoidoscopy versus colonoscopy.** The American Cancer Society used to recommend periodic flexible sigmoidoscopies in all patients over the age of 50 for colorectal cancer screening. That has changed, and now a complete colonoscopy is recommended for patients over the age of 50. Thirty percent of all patients over 50 will have benign, precancerous polyps at colonoscopy that the gastroenterologist will routinely remove during the procedure. You will be then asked to return every three to five years for a follow-up colonoscopy to ensure that the polyps have not returned. If the doctor performing your colonoscopy is less experienced, they may not have the training or ability to remove the polyps will require you to have a second costly procedure with a specialist. Because of how complex this operation is, colonoscopies should be performed only by a board-certified gastroenterologist.

- **Electrocardiogram (ECG or EKG).** Everyone 40 years and older should have a baseline EKG (footnote). This is also the case if you or your family has a history of cardiovascular problems. It is appropriate to test after you have taken any drugs that may influence your heartbeat. If you have remained clinically stable after having symptoms such as chest pain, chest pressure, shortness of breath, dizziness, or an irregular heartbeat and the doctor has ruled out any serious health issues, you should not be tested more than once a year, unless you already have been identified as having cardiac disease.

- **Stress test.** Anyone who is at risk for heart disease or even mild hypertension should probably have a stress test. It should be performed by a board-certified cardiologist, because if it is done by someone who is not experienced with the guidelines, you might get a false positive. A more complicated stress test is more costly and may actually pose a risk for someone who actually has a complication. These indications can be found on www.acc.org.
- **Sonogram.** The person that you choose to interpret the sonogram depends on the area you are identifying. It should be someone in that specialty because only they will know what they are looking for and in the end it will cost you less.

The U.S. Preventive Services Task Force, in fact, has criticized doctors for spending their time on questionable tests instead of counseling people about the harmful effects of smoking, lack of exercise, and other lifestyle risks. The only tests the task force recommended were:

- **Periodic blood pressure checkups for for all adults.** High blood pressure is a leading risk factor for coronary heart disease, stroke, renal disease, and heart attacks.
- **Total blood cholesterol measurement for men between the ages of 35 and 65 and women 45 to 65.** High cholesterol is a risk factor for heart disease. The task force did not specify how often the tests should be held.
- **Screening for colorectal cancer for individuals over 50.** The task force recommended testing by examining stools for the presence of blood, or through sigmoidoscopy. Colorectal cancer is common in the United States.
- **Mammogram for women between 50 and 69.** This x-ray to detect the early signs of breast cancer should be conducted every one or two years.
- **The Pap smear for sexually active women.** This test screens for cervical cancer and should be done once every three years.
- **Vision tests for children, before entering school, and for the elderly.**
- **Tests for elderly people (or those with specific complaints) to assess hearing loss.**

Another simple but helpful test screens for glaucoma, which may cause blindness (by measuring intraocular pressure). The roles and benefits of the following tests are still unclear:

- Routine blood sugar testing (to screen for diabetes)
- Testing for thyroid hormones in the blood (to screen for thyroid disease)
- Bone densitometry testing of menopausal women (to screen for osteoporosis)

Even the experts have differing recommendations. For example, there is currently a major controversy as to whether mammogram testing should begin at the age of 40 or 50. There are far more false positives among younger women, possibly because women in the 40 to 50 age group have denser breasts than those over 50. Recent studies prove that young women will stand a 50 percent chance of receiving a false positive during 10 years of annual mammograms. Because of this, some women endure intense anxiety and sometimes disfiguring biopsies before learning that they don't even have cancer.

In order to keep this from happening to you, it's vital that you know your medical history. That means not only your own but that of your family (your siblings, parents, grandparents, and even great-grandparents). Just knowing what is in your family's health history will help you avoid unnecessary preventive screenings. See Appendix D for a health history worksheet.

There is another controversy around screening for prostate cancer (either by rectal examination or through a blood test). The PSA (prostate specific antigen) blood test measures the level of a specific protein in your blood that can indicate cancer and other prostate abnormalities. The drawback here is that elevated levels do not mean you have prostate cancer, and in fact, about 20 percent of the time when the levels are elevated, it may not mean you have prostate cancer; however, if the levels are minimally elevated, the doctor might simply repeat the test. On the other hand, if these PSA levels are significantly elevated, you may be asked to have a prostate biopsy and perhaps even surgery to remove your prostate altogether. There are many ill effects from widespread screening for prostate cancer, including:

- A large number of false positives
- Unnecessary biopsies

Men

Screening Tests	Ages 18–39	Ages 40–49	Ages 50–64	Ages 65 and Older
General Health: Full checkup, including weight and height	Typically every 3 years. Discuss with your doctor or nurse.	Typically every 2 years. Discuss with your doctor or nurse.	Typically every year. Discuss with your doctor or nurse.	Typically every year. Discuss with your doctor or nurse.
Heart Health: Blood pressure test	At least every 2 years (preferably every year) starting at the age of 30 if your initial results are normal and have no history of heart or vascular disease.	At least every 2 years	Every year.	Every year.
Cholesterol test	Start at age 20, if you smoke, have diabetes, or if heart disease runs in your family, otherwise have the initial test at 20, and if you are normal and have none of the before-mentioned, at least every 5 years starting at 35. Discuss with your doctor or nurse.	Discuss with your doctor or nurse.	Discuss with your doctor or nurse.	Discuss with your doctor or nurse.
Electrocardiogram (EKG)	Initial EKG should be at 30.	Typically every 4 years. Discuss with your doctor or nurse.	Typically every 3 years. Discuss with your doctor or nurse.	Tpically every 3 years. Discuss with your doctor or nurse.
Diabetes: Blood sugar test	Have a test to screen for diabetes if you have high blood pressure or high cholesterol. Be sure to discuss with your doctor or nurse.	Start at age 45, then every 3 years.	Every 3 years.	Every 3 years.

Screening Tests	Ages 18–39	Ages 40–49	Ages 50–64	Ages 65 and Older
Glaucoma screening	At least once and for men at high risk, every 3-5 years.	Every 2-4 years.	Every 2-4 years.	Every 1-2 years.
Urinalysis	Specifically for cholesterol, diabetes, kidney and thyroid dysfunction every 3 years.	Every 2-3 years.	Every 2-3 years.	Every 2-3 years.
Prostate Health: Digital Rectal Exam (DRE)		Discuss with your doctor or nurse.	Discuss with your doctor or nurse.	Discuss with your doctor or nurse.
Prostate-Specific Antigen (PSA) (blood test)		Discuss with your doctor ornurse. Recommended for African-American men and men with a family history of prostate cancer at 40 years of age.	Every year.	Every year.
Reproductive Health: Testicular exam	Monthly self-exam; and part of a general checkup.	Monthly self-exam; and part of a general checkup.	Monthly self-exam; and part of a general checkup.	Monthly self-exam; and part of a general checkup.
Chlamydia test	Discuss with your doctor or nurse.	Discuss with your doctor or nurse.	Discuss with your doctor or nurse.	Discuss with your doctor or nurse.
Testosterone screening			Discuss with your doctor or nurse.	Discuss with your doctor or nurse.
Sexually Trnasmitted Disease (STD) tests	Both partners should get tested for STDs, including HIV, before initiating sexual intercourse.	Both partners should get tested for STDs, including HIV, before initiating sexual intercourse.	Both partners should get tested for STDs, including HIV, before initiating sexual intercourse.	Both partners should get tested for STDs, including HIV, before initiating sexual intercourse.

Men (continued)

Screening Tests	Ages 18–39	Ages 40–49	Ages 50–64	Ages 65 and Older
Colorectal Health: Fecal occult blood test/Hemoccult			Yearly.	Yearly.
Flexible Sigmoidoscopy (with fecal occult blood test is preferred)			Every 5 years (if not having a colonoscopy)	Every 5 years (if not having a colonoscopy)
Double Contrast Barium Enema (DCBE)			Every 5-10 years (if not having a colonoscopy or sigmoidoscopy)	Every 5-10 years (if not having a colonoscopy or sigmoidoscopy)
Colonoscopy			Every 10 years and every 3 years if you are at high risk.	Every 10 years and every 3 years if you are at high risk.
Rectal exam	Discuss with your doctor or nurse.	Discuss with your doctor or nurse.	Every 5-10 years with each screening (sigmoidoscopy, colonoscopy, or DCBE)	Every 5-10 years with each screening (sigmoidoscopy, colonoscopy, or DCBE)
Eye and Ear Health: Eye exam	Get your eyes checked if you have problems or visual changes.	Every 2-4 years.	Every 2-4 years.	Every 1-2 years.
Hearing test	Starting at age 18, then every 10 years.	Every 10 years.	Discuss with your doctor or nurse.	Discuss with your doctor or nurse.
Skin Health: Mole exam	Monthly mole self-exam; by a doctor every 3 years, starting at age 20.	Monthly mole self-exam; by a doctor every year.	Monthly mole self-exam; by a doctor every year.	Monthly mole self-exam; by a doctor every year.
Tuberculosis skin test	Every 5 years.	Every 5 years.	Typically every year.	Typically every year.

Screening Tests	Ages 18–39	Ages 40–49	Ages 50–64	Ages 65 and Older
Oral Health: Dental exam	One to two times every year.	One to two times every year.	One to two times every year.	One to two times every year.
Immunizations: Influenza vaccine	Discuss with your doctor or nurse.	Discuss with your doctor or nurse.	Yearly.	Yearly.
Pneumococcal vaccine				One time only; however, you may need it earlier if you have certain health problems, such as lung disease.
Hepatitis B	Discuss with your doctor or nurse.	Discuss with your doctor or nurse.	Discuss with your doctor or nurse.	Discuss with your doctor or nurse.
Tetanus-Diphtheria Booster vaccine	Every 10 years.	Every 10 years.	Every 10 years.	Every 10 years.
X-rays: Chest Xray			Discuss with your doctor or nurse. Especially if you were a smoker.	Discuss with your doctor or nurse. Especially if you were a smoker.
Bone Health Screening:			About 60 years of age. Discuss with your doctor or nurse.	
Aspirin:	Discuss with your doctor or nurse if you have high blood pressure, high cholesterol, diabetes, or if you smoke.	Discuss with yuor doctor or nurse about taking aspirin to prevent heart disease.	Discuss with your doctor or nurse about taking aspirin to prevent heart disease.	Discuss with your doctor or nurse about taking aspirin to prevent heart disease.

Women

Screening Tests	Ages 18–39	Ages 40–49	Ages 50–64	Ages 65 and Older
General Health: Full checkup, including weight and height	Discuss with your doctor or nurse.	Discuss with your doctor or nurse.	Discuss with your doctor or nurse.	Discuss with your doctor or nurse.
Thyroid test (TSH)	Start at age 35, then every 5 years.	Every 5 years.	Every 5 years.	Every 5 years.
Heart Health: Blood pressure test	At least every 2 years: age 30 for Caucasians, and age 25 for African Americans.	At least every 2 years.	At least every 2 years.	At least every 2 years.
Cholesterol test	Start at age 20, if you smoke, have diabetes,, or if heart disease runs in your family. Discuss with your doctor or nurse.	Start at the age of 45 every year. Discuss with your doctor or nurse.	Every year. Discuss with your doctor or nurse.	Every year. Discuss with your doctor or nurse.
Bone Health: Bone mineral density test		Discuss with your doctor or nurse, especially if you have a family history of osteoporosis (thinning of the bones).	Discuss with your doctor or nurse. If you are between the ages of 60 and 64 and weigh 154 lbs. or less, talk to your doctor about whether you should be tested.	Get a bone mineral density test at least once. Talk to your doctor or nurse about repeat testing.
Diabetes: Blood sugar test	Discuss with your doctor or nurse. Screen for diabetes if you have high blood pressure or high cholesterol at age 25.	Start at age 45, then every 3 years.	Every 3 years.	Every 3 years.

Screening Tests	Ages 18–39	Ages 40–49	Ages 50–64	Ages 65 and Older
Breast Health: Mammogram (x-ray of breast)		Every 1-2 years. Discuss with your doctor or nurse.	Every 1-2 years. Discuss with your doctor or nurse.	Every 1-2 years. Discuss with your doctor or nurse.
Reproductive Health: Pap test & pelvic exam	Every 1-3 years if you have been sexually active or are older than 21.	Every 1-3 years.	Every 1-3 years.	Discuss with your doctor or nurse.
Chlamydia test	If sexually active, yearly until age 25. Ages 26-39, if you are at high risk for chlamydia or other STDs, you may need this test.	If you are at high risk for chlamydia or other sexually transmitted diseases (STDs) you may need this test.	If you are at high risk for chlamydia or other sexually transmitted diseases (STDs) you may need this test.	If you are at high risk for chlamydia or other sexually transmitted diseases (STDs) you may need this test.
Sexually Transmitted Disease (STD) tests	Both partners should get tested for STDs, including HIV, before initiating sexual intercourse.	Both partners should get tested for STDs, including HIV, before initiating sexual intercourse.	Both partners should get tested for STDs, including HIV, before initiating sexual intercourse.	Both partners should get tested for STDs, including HIV, before initiating sexual intercourse.
Colorectal Health: Colorectal Cancer Tests			Your doctor can help you decide which test is right for you.	Discuss with your doctor or nurse.
Aspirin:		Discuss with your doctor or nurse about taking aspirin to prevent heart disease if you are older than 45 and have high blood pressure, high cholesterol diabetes, or if you smoke.	Discuss with your doctor or nurse about taking aspirin to prevent heart disease.	Discuss with your doctor or nurse about taking aspirin to prevent heart disease.

Women (continued)

Screening Tests	Ages 18–39	Ages 40–49	Ages 50–64	Ages 65 and Older
Immunizations: Influenza vaccine	Discuss with your doctor or nurse.	Discuss with your doctor or nurse.	Yearly.	Yearly.
Pneumococcal vaccine				One time only; however, you may need it earlier if you have certain health problems, such as lung disease.
Tetanus-Diphtheria Booster vaccine	Every 10 years.	Every 10 years.	Every 10 years.	Every 10 years.
Hepatitis B	Discuss with your doctor or nurse.	Discuss with your doctor or nurse.	Discuss with your doctor or nurse.	Discuss with your doctor or nurse.

• Harmful side effects of aggressive treatments for slowly growing cancers (which might never have become dangerous and could have been left alone)

The Task Force suggests that doctor's time would be more productive if they spent it discussing unhealthy behavior patterns with their patients. They believe that your doctor can do far more for you by convincing you to stop smoking than by subjecting you to multiple tests or by prescribing many pills with shady results.

The question you need the answer to is this: What can you do to get the maximum benefits from your medical checkup?

First, you do not need to go for a checkup every year. If you are healthy, have no symptoms, and are in your 20s or 30s, you can safely have a physical only once every two to five years. However, this checkup should be exhaustive. When you go in, take all your relevant medical records, for instance, your medical and family history and all the medications you are taking (or have taken). Tell your doctor details about your lifestyle. Your doctor should talk to you and listen to you during your checkup, since disease prevention is as important as detection.

If you do not have any indicative symptoms, you do not need a chest x-ray, electrocardiogram, or complete blood work. These do not provide your doctor with any clinically useful information. Many people believe "the more tests, the better the outcome." They are attracted to expensive checkup packages that offer more tests ("better value for money"). Please be forewarned: This is not true. A cost-effective checkup can be very simple and should include the following and no more:

- A physical examination measuring your height, weight, pulse, and blood pressure
- Blood tests for cholesterol
- Screening for colorectal cancer

For women, the physical should also include a Pap smear and a screening for breast cancer.

If your health insurance doesn't provide you adequate coverage, or if you don't have any health insurance coverage at all, you may want to look into free health screenings. Local clinics and hospitals often provide a variety of screenings, such as blood pressure, cholesterol, and mammograms. Some of these tests can be given to you for virtually nothing at your local community health center—depending on your income. To locate the center closest to you, call INFOLINE at 211, which is similar to dialing 411 for information, except that this is to find the closest clinic in your area, or your local health department by searching for the number in the blue pages of your phonebook. Some of these centers offer free or low-cost breast and cervical cancer screens and treatments for women as well as immunizations, blood pressure, cholesterol screenings, and more.

Schools specializing in dental teaching, and other schools teaching medical services, might also offer free or low-cost services such as dental cleaning. If you have children, check your school to see if they have a health center or if they get regular visits from a medical or dental van. College students should check with their school to find if they get free or reduced-cost care.

While it is true that your doctor is your most valuable source of information, do not forget about other resources like books, libraries, CDs, and the Internet. It's not always easy to collect information, but patience and persistence can help you find precisely what you're looking for. You should be able to trust your doctor, but it's also a good idea to be able to independently confirm his advice. For example, if your doctor recommends surgery and you double-check and discover that his judgment is right, you will have even more confidence in him. Doing your homework will allow you to use your time with your doctor well spent, and will allow you to ask focused questions about your health problems.

CHAPTER 14

How to Read Your Medical Bill

Understand Your Hospital Medical Records

Medical bills are often confusing. In order to understand how to read your medical bill, you first must understand where your charges originate. For example, as soon as you make an initial appointment for the clinic or hospital, the bill begins and your medical record is created.

What are your medical records? These can be voluminous documents associated with your care, which can be difficult for the nonclinician to understand. These documents include papers, reports, forms, x-rays, and charts in no specific order. Often the records do not correlate well with the bill received, and it would be in your best interest to review them with your doctor or another medical professional. This can clarify details of charges on the bill which are in medical terms and which you do not recognize. If you request copies of the record, you will usually be charged; however, once you understand the structure of these records, you can comprehend the details of your billing a little more easily. Remember: just because you don't recognize the charge doesn't mean it was not done. So save yourself some embarrassment and review it with a professional before pursuing a complaint.

Documents Common to Most Health Records

- The identification sheet is a form that originates at the time of admission. This form lists your name, address, and telephone number.

- The document on History and Physical/Clinical Findings describes factors such as:
  - Any major illnesses and surgeries you have had
  - Any significant family history of disease
  - Your health habits
  - Current medications.
  - Your height, weight, blood pressure, pulse, respiration rate, any particular symptoms you may have described, and details of your physical examination.
- Progress Notes are notes made by the doctors, nurses, and therapists caring for you that reflect your response to treatment and their observations and plans for continued treatment.
- Consultation is an opinion about your condition made by a physician other than your primary care physician. Sometimes, a consultation is performed because your physician needs the advice and counsel of another physician. At other times, a consultation occurs when you yourself request a second opinion.
- Physician's Orders are contained in a document that records your physician's directions regarding your medications, tests, diet and treatments.
- Imaging and X-ray Reports are documents describing x-ray results, mammograms, ultrasounds, or scans. The actual films are usually stored in the radiology or imaging departments.
- Electrocardiogram (ECG, EKG) Reports.
- Lab Reports describe the results of tests conducted on blood, sputum, urine and other body fluids. Common examples would include a urinalysis, complete blood count (CBC), cholesterol level, and throat culture.
- Authorization Forms include copies of consents for admission, treatment and surgery.
- The Operative Report is a document describing the surgery performed and gives the names of the surgeons and assistants involved.
- The Anesthesia Report is a form documenting the preoperative medication, anesthesia given, and the response to anesthesia during surgery.

- The Pathology Report describes tissue removed during an operation (if any) and gives a diagnosis based on the examination of that tissue.
- The Graphic Sheet is generally a graph used to plot your temperature, pulse, respiration, and blood pressure over a particular period of time.
- The Discharge Summary presents a concise account of your stay, which includes the following information: the reason for admission; the significant findings from tests; the procedures performed; the therapies provided; the response to treatment; the condition during discharge; and instructions for medications, activity, diet, and follow-up care.

All of the above charges are divided into two major components. They are the professional and the technical components of your medical bill. The professional component is the actual service or the interpretation of the result of a test usually performed by a doctor. The technical component is the equipment and the technician performing the test. So when you get a medical bill and it says "pelvic x-ray," this is considered the technical component. This does not include the interpretation of the x-ray, such as if a fracture was found by the radiologist. The interpretation of the x-ray will be charged on a separate bill known as the "professional component." These bills might arrive in your mailbox months apart from each other, which is why it is important to get a summAry of all procedures performed before leaving the facility. This way you can know what bills to expect.

When you receive the bills, check to make sure they accurately reflect the procedures you have undergone and take into account any applicable insurance coverage you may have. Some errors, such as wrong computer codes, are common, and you may be billed for healthcare you never received. Contact the appropriate billing office if you think you've found a mistake. If you've received an explanation of benefits from your insurance company that you believe is wrong, ask the company to review your claim.

It is imperative that you view these records and question your treatment and condition for several reasons; you are being charged, you have a right to know what is being procedures/treatments are being performed and why, and to verify that you are being told what is being written in your medical record. Some nurses and doctors still do not know that patients have the right to see their own medical records. To avoid being the ictim of a misinformed medical professional, it is vital that you know your rights. In fact, some consumer advocates argue that it is a good idea for patients in a hospital to take a look at their own medical charts routinely, to make sure that the doctors and nurses have written down everything accurately; after all, medical notes can be inaccurate or incomplete, leading to confusion in the future.

How do you go about getting copies of your records? Simple: just ask your doctor or hospital and sign a records release! Remember that you have a legal right to your medical record, and while technically the documents belong to the doctor or hospital; in most cases, the information about you belongs to you. Remember, the hospital may charge you for making copies, and you will need to pay the required amount.

While your records are very helpful in improving the quality of your medical care, do not forget that they can also prove extremely important in case you are unhappy with the care you received. If you need to complain about your doctor or hospital, the records can be used to support your claim, even for a discount in you bill. These days, most hospitals have "patient advocacy" groups that will help with these issues and are sure that they are properly resolved before it is too late. Often times, if an unanticipated complication occurs in the course of your care, the hospital will gladly give a discount rather than face a potential malpractice claim.

The same holds true if you do not understand why something was done or not done. You have a right to ask for an explanation and should be given one you can understand. for example, due to the shortage of nursing staff, many hospitals place Foley catheters in their elderly patients for the convenience of the staff (i.e., nurses do not have to attend to the patient as much because now, if a patient needs to urinate, he or she just goes through a tube instead of calling a nurse for assistance). As a patient, you are being charged for the Foley catheter as well as the catheterization (both technical fees). If you are not satisfied with the explanation given by the nurse, be sure to ask a doctor *before* it becomes a procedure and equipment charge on your bill!

In addition, keep in mind that you are charged for every meal, even if you do not request it or missed it. So if you feel the need to skip a meal, be sure the nurse documents that you requested no meal and be sure it does not show up on your bill months later. You will likely forget the details of the charges on your bill, so it is important to *write it down* and document your concerns to the hospital administration at the time of the hospitalization. The hospital medical bill can take months to arrive, long after your insurance has paid its part of the bill.

Also, keep in mind that every doctor who examines you while you are staying in the hospital will be charging you, which is why it is important to maintain a good relationship with your primary care physician. If he or she agrees that no other physician needs to see you, be sure you are not charged. Even the doctor who pops his head in to ask how you are doing and orders some meds will charge for the visit. Your primary care doctor should let you know when a specialist or another physician is needed.

Not only are medical records a vital source of information for the patient, but they also provide imperative information to the insurance companies when you need to claim reimbursement for expenses for medical treatment from your insurance company. If procedures/treatments are not being documented, or even documented appropriately, it may cost you more in the end.

To put the importance of your medical records into perspective, remember that records serve many purposes. For instance, these records provide:

- The basis for planning your care and treatment
- A means of communication among the many health professionals who contribute to your care
- Basic data for health research and planning
- Verification of services and treatment covered by your insurance.
- A legal document describing the care you receive

Most important, pay particular attention to the diagnosis the doctor writes down in your record to be sure it corresponds with your treatment. for example, if the reason you are admitted is for chest pain, and in the course of testing it is discovered that you have iron-deficiency anemia and require colonoscopy/upper endoscopy, etc., make sure the anemia diagnosis is clearly outlined as urgent and the in-hospital evaluation necessary. Otherwise your insurance company may deny payment for the inpatient work up, and you may get stuck with the bill. Unfortunately, most insurance companies have a protocol of treatments they expect the doctor to follow in order to get reimbursed. If the doctor prescribes a different treatment or set of tests than the insurance carrier is not used to seeing, it is likely you will not get reimbursed. This is why it is better to catch it before it becomes an issue by reviewing your record as soon as it becomes available. If this happens, your doctor should have an explanation and be able to write a letter on your behalf to your insurance company stating the reasons the treatment was necessary based on your diagnosis. Subsequently, reimbursement should not be a problem. If this happens more than once, it may be time to get a new insurance policy.

On the other hand, hospital coding specialists will try to create a higher-billing CPT code that will match one of your diagnoses. Essentially, every diagnosis is matched to a code, and that code signifies a dollar amount that you or your insurance will be paying. The higher the billing code, the more the hospital gets paid, regardless of how many days you stay in the hospital. For example, an "in-and-out urine catheterization" has a code that charges less than one third the cost of the placement of a Foley catheter, which carries a nursing procedural fee and an equipment fee. So it is imperative to match the hospital billing codes with what was actually was performed and be sure they correlate precisely. Often discrepancies occur and can be challenged only if you have documented exatly what really transpired. This can be painstaking and difficult to do but it can save thousands in the long run. For some unclear reason, hospitals usually take months to up to a year to send patients a final, itemized bill. By this time, most patients have forgotten details of the hospital stay and do not recall what specifically should or should not appear on the bill. If this occurs purposefully, it can be termed *delayed price escalation* and is dependent on the amnesia of the patient being "price-gouged."

In order to avoid all chaos before it begins, be sure you request an itemized bill so you can check it against your medical records before you leave the hospital or clinic. Making sure that all the charges on your hospital bill are justified and reasonable is a formidable undertaking. But it can be easier if you know what to look for. Please keep in mind that it may take a few days, or even weeks for the clinic/hospital to produce the itemized bill and records due to the fact there is a process of coding that must happen in order for the doctor and his staff to be paid for his work. Ask nicely when you should expect to receive these documents and from whom as well as a contact number and name in case you do not receive the documents within the promised time.

When you finally receive the itemized bill, pay special attention to the most common areas of overcharges and errors, plus any irregularities in your medical records and itemized bill, for example:

- **Duplicate billing:** Make sure you haven't been charged twice for the same service, supplies, or medications.
- **Duplication of tests:** Be sure to ask the doctor the kind and frequency of blood tests, x-rays, and medical procedures you will have to undergo.
- **Number of days in hospital:** Check the dates of your admission and discharge. Were you charged for the discharge day? Most hospitals will charge for admission day, but not for day of discharge.
- **Incorrect room charges:** If you were in a semi-private room, make sure you're not being charged for a private one.
- **Operating room time:** It's not uncommon for hospitals to bill for more time than you actually used. Compare the charge with your anesthesiologist's records.
- **Upcoding:** Hospitals often shift the charge for a lower-cost service or medication to one that's more costly. For example, a doctor orders a generic drug, but the patient is charged for a pricier brand name.
- **Keystroke error:** A computer operator accidentally hits the wrong key on a keyboard. It can cost you hundreds of dollars and result in an incorrect charge for a service you didn't get.
- **Canceled work:** Your physician ordered an expensive test and then canceled it, but you were charged anyway.
- **Services never rendered:** Did you get every service, treatment, and medication for which you are being billed? Here's where your log will come in handy.
- **Erroneous charges:** Such as $90 charged for a 70-cent IV or $129 for a "mucous recovery system" otherwise known as a box of Kleenex.

It seems that hospitals discourage you from examining your bills. Please be proactive and don't leave it up to the insurance companies. If your hospitalization isn't for an emergency, check your insurance policy to find out just what it will cover and how much it will pay. Be sure to carefully review the section on "exceptions and exclusions."

It will tell you what your plan will not cover. To avoid problems, consider doing the following:

- Phone the hospital's billing department and ask them what you will be charged for the room and what the room charges cover. If tissues aren't included, for example, bring your own.
- Ask your doctor to estimate your cost of treatment. Also, ask if you can bring your regular prescriptions from home to avoid paying for medications administered at the hospital.
- Make sure that everyone who will be treating you—the surgeon, anesthesiologist, radiologist, pathologist, etc.—participates in your insurance plan.
- If you can, keep your own log of tests, medications, and treatments. If you are not able to, ask a friend or loved one to do it for you.
- At some point you will receive an explanation of benefits (EOB), also explained in Chapter 5, from your insurance company (if you're on Medicare, you will receive a summary notice). It will say, "This is not a bill." Don't toss it into the trash. Examine it. It will tell you how much the hospital is charging, what your insurance plan will cover, and what you will have to pay out of your own pocket in deductibles and copayments.
- Never pay your bill before leaving the hospital—even if you're told that it's required.
- When you get your bill, read it carefully. Compare it to the log you made, to the EOB, and to the estimate of costs you requested before you were admitted.
- If there are items you don't understand, call the billing department and your insurer, and ask them to explain. Don't accept bills that use terms such as "lab fees" or "miscellaneous fees." Demand an itemization. If you don't get satisfaction from the hospital billing department—and you probably won't—appeal in writing to the hospital administrator or patient ombudsman. Most hospitals have "patient advocacy programs" these days that can help you with this.
- Always ask for an itemized bill as well as your medical records to confirm whether or not you received the treatments and medications you've been billed for. Every state now requires hospitals to provide itemized bills.

Should I Ignore My Bill?

As described in some of the other chapters, as soon as a clinician interacts with you, the billing process will begin; however, depending on your healthcare insurance, income status, bill and resources, your final bill may be negotiable, but first you need to make sure you take the right steps.

First of all, keep in mind that if your case involves a car accident or a worker's compensation issue, by law, the other party will be billed first, and thus you will have an extended period of time to figure out how you are going to pay your bill before you are sent to collection. In the past, many hospitals "wrote off" unpaid medical bills because the attorneys' fees were not worth the amount the hospitals would collect in the end; however, more and more hospitals have hired collection attorneys on a contingency basis so that they receive a percentage of what they find in the unpaid patient's assets.

Typically, the patient will receive at least three statements from the facility before they decide to either write the bill off or file a legal judgment against a patient who has decided not to pay a bill. If you fall into the latter of the two categories, this will eventually go on your credit history and, most of the time, will not show up until you try to make a large purchase, such as a house. In the meantime, the hospital writes both situations off as a "bad debt" if no action takes place in about six months.

On the other hand, if you refuse to pay a bill due to what you perceive is a billing mistake, call the billing department immediately and ask for an itemization of your bill, including a pharmaceutical itemization. At this time, it would be wise to call the patient advocacy group or customer service department to let them know what steps you are taking and why so they can document you have been proactive and maybe they can help facilitate the process for you. You should also want to call the charge nurse or the nursing director and ask for a copy of your medical records. This, as we described earlier in the book is the "technical" part of the bill. Typically, it should take the healthcare facility anywhere from 72 to 96 hours or maybe even a week depending how busy the hospital is to locate all your records and make copies.

At this point you still need to receive a copy of the "professional" part of the bill, which will include all the "readings" done, such as the pathologist, radiologist, techs, and any physicians that gave an opinion of diagnosis on your case.

After all this has been done, keep in mind that you still need to talk to your attending physician or primary care physician who orchestrated your stay in the healthcare facility regarding the professional charges alone. It may take your physician a few days to get back to you due to his workoad, but his staff should be able to explain applicable charges and if you have a good relationship with your physician, you may be able to negotiate a lower rate for his services. Some patient advocacy groups may even offer to call all the "professional" components of your bill and negotiate for you, depending on your financial situation.

Always remember that people who work in the healthcare industry care about people, so if you are pleasant and honest, they will usually be more than willing to help.

CHAPTER 15

EVERYDAY WAYS TO LOWER YOUR HEALTHCARE BILLS

PRESCRIPTION DRUGS ARE AN ever-increasing cost of health care. Being an informed consumer about the choice and cost of medications can help save money for you and your family. This chapter suggests several ways to help you lower the cost of prescription medications, as well as some other everyday savings tips that you may not be aware of. You should discuss these options with your doctor or pharmacist to make sure they are right for you. One of the best ways to save dollars is to pay attention to where your pennies go.

Prescription Drugs

Although there are no foul-proof methods when it comes to saving money on prescription drugs, here are some questions that you may ask yourself that may uncover some options that may help you reduce your expenses. Ask yourself these twelve questions:

1. Does your insurance cover the prescriptions you need?
2. Will samples be sufficient? (In other words, will this prescription need many refills or will you only need a few pills?)
3. Do you qualify for a pharmaceutical company's drug assistance program?
4. Do you qualify for a state program?

5. Can your brand name drugs be substituted for a less expensive generic version?
6. Are over-the-counter drugs available?
7. Is one pharmacy less expensive than another pharmacy?
8. Is mail order or bulk buying an option?
9. Is an Internet or discount drug program available?
10. Can cutting your pills save you money?
11. Can importing drugs save you money?
12. Does your physician have a good relationship with a local pharmacy/pharmacist?

Does Your Insurance Cover the Prescriptions You Need?

Some people make the mistake of purchasing health insurance that does not have a drug plan. Be sure to read the drug benefits under the insurance plan you choose. Call your insurance plan directly and ask what pharmaceuticals they may cover. You can consult with your primary care physician to find out which insurance company has the most flexible drug plan in your area.

If you find out your insurance doesn't cover the exact medication you are looking for, call your doctor right away (or the pharmacist can call for you) to substitute the drug with something that is comparable and covered.

You may want to check if your insurance company allows you more than a months worth of prescriptions at a time. This may be able to save you money, as there is a per-ticket fee for every prescription (to pay for the bottle, label, sack, paperwork, etc), so getting several months at once (if feasible) can remove some of the per-ticket fees if you don't have a flat co-pay. If you have a flat co-pay, you may be able to get more than one month (usually 3 months) and avoid extra payment. This depends on your insurer, so don't blame the pharmacist.

Will Samples Be Sufficient?

If you have an acute condition, such as a peptic ulcer, you may be able to ask your doctor for assistance in obtaining samples. Pharmaceutical companies will sometimes provide drugs samples to give to those who are unable to wait to have a prescription filled. It's designed to allow you to start a new drug to see if it may work before committing to a long term prescription.

If your doctor gives you a prescription for something minor like acute pain or minor infection, and you cannot afford it, ask him or her for free samples. They may have enough for your whole treatment, or just enough to get you started and then you can get the rest of what you need at the pharmacy. It's against the law to charge for samples. If your physician doesn't know how much a prescription should cost, ask his office staff to call the local pharmacy while you are there to check their prices. This is often a great eye opener for most physicians. Cipro 500mg (an antibiotic) can run over $150 for a 10 day course in our area and there are no generic substitutes. If you can't afford the drug your doctor suggests to you, insist on something else. It only works if you can afford to take it! Ask if they carry any samples of the drug. Offices and hospitals receive samples for free from the drug companies so don't be bashful about taking them.

In recent years, drug vouchers have become been more commonplace than samples. The drug voucher is a coupon for the drug that you take to the pharmacy for free medication. The drug company later reimburses the pharmacy for their costs.

Do You Qualify For a Pharmaceutical Company's Drug Assistance Program?

Most major pharmaceutical companies participate in a program or programs that are designed to assist you pay for their medication. Each company has their own criteria, but it's usually your insurance coverage and income. If you can demonstrate true financial hardship and can qualify for one of their programs, most companies will provide their drug at no charge.

Pfizer's patient assistance program is called "Connection to Care." If you are single and your total household income is $19,000 or less per year, or married with a total household income of $31,000 or less a year, and do not have health insurance, Pfizer will send you a three-month supply of medication to your health care provider. For more information on this program, you can call 1-800-707-8990. Pfizer also includes other uninsured Americans regardless of their income through programs like "Pfizer Friends," which offers steep discounts on pharmaceuticals. For more information, you can call 1-866-706-2400.

Novartis offers free 30, 90, and 180 day supplies if you are a U.S resident, meet the income requirements, and have no prescription drug coverage. You must call 1-800-277-2254 to find out if you qualify.

GlaxoSmithKline has a program specific to oncology patients in need of their pharmaceuticals. Their website is www.commitmenttoacess.gsk.com, or you can call 1-866-265-6491 directly. Their general patient assistance program can be found at www.bridgestoaccess.gsk.com or at 1-800-699-3806.

Eli Lilly has two programs. Medicare recipients are offered Lilly products at $12 a month, which must be purchased at your local pharmacy. To qualify, you must have no other prescription drug coverage and an individual annual income below $18,000, or a household income below $24,000. For more information, go online at www.lillyanswers .com or call 1-877-795-4559. If you do not qualify for Medicare benefits, the Lilly Cares program is free of charge for qualifying U.S. residents who need temporary assistance in obtaining their Lilly or Dista medications. Go to www.lilly-cares.com to find out if you qualify or call 1-800-545-6962.

Some pharmaceutical companies decided to form an alliance and now offer 25 to 40 percent and sometimes more on over 275 prescription drugs and products as well as some generic drugs at participating pharmacies. This program is called Together Rx Access. For more information on which pharmaceutical companies are participating and the type of discounts that can be expected, go to www.TogetherRxAccess.com or call 1-800-444-4106.

Partnership for Prescription Assistance is a one-stop-shop that, if you qualify, will help you get the medicines they need through the public or private program that's right for them. As of now, 45 pharmaceutical companies provide this company with information for over 150 programs. To find out more information about participating companies, you may go online to https://www.pparx.org/Intro.php or call 1-888-477-2669. Not all companies and programs may be up dated, so be sure to identify the manufacturer of your particular prescription and call them directly to find out what programs they may be offering that you may qualify for. Your doctor should be able to help you figure out the manufacturer.

Do You Qualify For A State Program?

All states have programs that are designed to both help those who have financial difficulties as well as those who have specific diseases or conditions that might be expensive to manage. To find out what programs exist and keep up with changes in your state, contact your state Department of Health, Medicaid office, or go to the website of National Conference of State Legislators at www.ncsl.org/programs/health/ drugaid.htm. Another website that can help identify your state's medical assistance programs as well as pharmaceutical companies cooperating with these programs is the directory to the Medical Research Assistant at www.ec-online.net/Assistants/medresassistant.htm.

Every program will have a different set of requirements depending most of the time on your income level. Co-payments, deductibles, enrollment fees, and premiums may apply.

Can Your Brand Name Drugs Be Substituted For a Less Expensive Generic Version?

One of the most cost-saving methods in healthcare is actually the simplest. Generic drugs are chemically identical, but lower-cost version of a brand-name drug. The generic version of a drug becomes available when the brand-name drug's patent protection expires, or the FDA regulation and oversight is complete. In both cases, the cost is usually about half the price of the brand-name version.

All drugs have a generic name. When a pharmaceutical company first develops a new drug, it gives the drug a generic, or chemical, name. For example, the generic name for Tylenol is acetaminophen. The company then gives the drug a brand-name as part of its marketing plan. Generic drugs are just as regulated as brand name drugs—in fact, they are essentially the same drug. A website that will tell you the generic name for brand name drugs is www.drugdigest.org.

By federal law generic drugs have the same amount of active ingredients as brand name drugs. The sole difference is in the substances used to fill or pack them. If you have questions regarding them, you should discuss generics with your physician.

When you are dealing with generics, as well as with brand name drugs, you must always be aware of the side effects as well as your allergies. Everyone will react to drugs differently, so it is important to find the drug that works for you financially as well as therapeutically.

One important point to make: Any drug that requires you to maintain a level in you bloodstream (i.e. anti-seizure meds, anticoagulants, certain cardiac meds, and certain antipsychotic meds), must be maintained in the form you started. Switching from generic to brand name or vice versa could be fatal. The active components are the same, but your body may react differently with the filler and absorb not enough or too much of the active ingredient in the same dose. Some examples of drugs that you should not switch to its generic after taking are Coumadin (generic name: Warfarin Sodium), Synthroid (generic name: Levothyroxine Sodium), and Lanoxin (generic name: Digoxin). It's important to remember that this is not because of any flaw in the generic drugs. If your doctor writes you a prescription for Synthroid, Coumadin, or Lanoxin, make sure to request the generic the very first time, or you may be stuck taking the overpriced brand name until a dosage change is required.

When you are given the prescription sheet at your doctor's office, you should look to see if the box with the letters "DAW" or "dispense as written" is checked. If it is, the pharmacist is legally required to give you the brand drug and not the generic. If you notice this is checked, question your doctor as to if there is a generic drug available before you get to the pharmacy.

You should know your drug's price before going to your local pharmacy. Remember that pharmacies are in the market to make money, and prices from pharmacy to pharmacy may vary. Use the online calculator at www.excellusbcbs.com to help you determine the generic name of a particular drug, as well as the cost savings. This is not a comprehensive list, so you might have to do your own research to uncover the generic name. Use Costco's online Pharmacy (www.costco.com) to search for larger discounts on your generic drugs. Remember that some drugs, such as Ultracet, do not have a generic, but its partner drug Ultram, (generic name: Tramadol) does.

You should make sure, if you have any allergies, to ask your pharmacist about the ingredients in your medicine. There are sometimes several generic versions of a drug, with slightly different inactive ingredients, so there may be one that is just right for you. In any case, you should discuss with your physician the use of generic drugs and to what extent in order to avoid an even more expensive reaction.

Are Over-The-Counter Drugs Available?

Many drugs that were once prescriptions are now available over-the-counter. Be wary of the drugs that re-patent themselves with new names to keep you from changing to the less-expensive generic alternatives. A perfect example of this is Nexium (the new purple pill). While Nexium has the same basic molecule as Prilosec (an over-the-counter drug with a very affordable prescription generic, Omeprazole), Nexium has been advertised to be better. In truth, it is a mixture of left hand and right hand molecules and Prilosec contains only the right hand molecule. The study used in advertising to say Nexium works better actually compared the 40mg strength Nexium to 20mg strength Prilosec.

When you are pill shopping, remember to calculate the actual price per pill. Several stomach preparations, arthritis medications, and other drugs are now available over-the-counter in reduced strengths. There is also a tax incentive for purchasing over-the-counter if the drug can legally be written as a prescription. You may be able to write it off on your taxes, or even not have to pay sales tax. Ask your doctor for more information on this.

Is One Pharmacy Less Expensive Than Another Pharmacy?

It's important to shop around at different pharmacies for the lowest price but remember not to ignore their service and personalized attention. Not only do pharmacies differ in there charges, but some offer extra services such as a door-to-door delivery service. When you're price-checking, know the drug's name, dosage, and quantity needed. If you can't read the prescription, have your physician, his staff, or your pharmacist write it out for you.

It may make sense, after reviewing the prices, to start purchasing different drugs from different pharmacies, since there might be a vast difference in their prices. Be very careful if you do this—you could potentially lose track of your prescriptions.

You may also want to check into stores like Costco, Target, and Wal-Mart for even lower prices on generic drugs. Although stores like Costco traditional only open their discounts to members, some states require these store sell its drugs to non-members. Check the policy for your state. Many drugstore chains and some independent drugstores will match the lowest price available in your area for prescription drugs. Kmart will even match prices from the Internet and mail-order drug sellers. It pays to comparison shop and then ask your preferred pharmacy to match the lowest price. Not every store will do this.

If you are a senior, ask your pharmacy if they offer a senior citizen discount or other discounts from organizations you may belong to (such as AARP). Make sure to consider all of these discounts when cost-comparing various pharmacies.

Some pharmacies offer such steep discounts that it may be cheaper to buy the drug without insurance. If you have insurance, make sure you are paying your co-pay on the cheapest amount possible. For example, if you buy prenatal vitamins for $20 for 100 tablets, your insurance may cover a $7 co-pay for 30 days/pills. In other words, 90 tablets would cost $21, and without insurance, the same pills cost $20 for 100 tablets. Be sure you find out the base price of the medication before you hand in that card.

Double-check to see you still have refills available before you drive to the drugstore to save gas and time. The best way to check is to quickly call the drugstore, as the information on your bottle may be inaccurate (it could be expired or you may be looking at an older bottle).

Buy only one or two days worth of a new medication to see if it will work. If you need to change drugs after two days you have only bought the amount you have used. You can buy several pills at a time of any prescription, but then you are required to stick with that pharmacy until that prescription is completed (not including refills).

Is Mail Order or Bulk-Buying an Option?

The best option if you have a chronic illness is to purchase prescriptions in bulk or with a mail order service. AARP, Good SAM Travel Club, and Med-Express are just a few nationwide companies. These will save you money and most deliver directly to your door. To find a service that will work for you, call the company that produces the drug, found in the Physician's Desk Reference at your physicians office or at the pharmacy.

Is an Internet or Discount Drug Program Available?

Internet pharmacies are able to offer savings because of their centralized warehousing for fulfilling orders and the efficiencies of selling on such a large scale. An example of this is Drugstore.com of Bellevue, which saves its customers 20 percent to 30 percent on most prescriptions. It also allows you to sign up for e-mail notifications when a generic form of a drug you are taking has been approved by the government.

If you have drug coverage, this most likely will not help you, as you will be charged the same co-payment whether shopping online or at the local pharmacy. For seniors on Medicare and those who are uninsured, especially if you have a chronic illnesses, this is an excellent way to find cheaper drugs.

The biggest bargains come from Canada, thanks to government price controls. These price controls are why average discounts can be as much as 67 percent cheaper than U.S. prices. However, the Food and Drug Administration (FDA) now bans the cross-border shipment of drugs into the U.S.

It sends warning letters to overseas pharmacies and alerts the Customs Service to watch out for packages from them. They are also targeting overseas pharmacies that ship drugs to the U.S., but not if you are simply importing non-narcotic prescription drugs. Generally, you aren't risking prosecution unless you are ordering a controlled substance.

Besides for the legal issues, the FDA also warns that there are inadequate safeguards of the quality of overseas drugs. Here are a few guidelines to go through before ordering online:

- **Does the website look professional?** If the website looks like it was done by an amateur, chances are that the company is too. Information should be provided about drug interactions, as well as an address or phone number to a licensed pharmacist who can answer your questions. Test this by calling this number or sending an email to the company with a general question to see how they respond. Look for efficiency and accuracy. Their customer service policies should be posted, including what to do if a drug is recalled.

- **Is there a prescription requirement?** You should purchase only from sites that require prescriptions from a physician or other authorized health care provider—and who verify each prescription before dispensing the medication. This will allow your doctor a chance to confirm the medication will not interact with another medication you are on. It will also give you a fax number or address so you can give them your prescription information. Their written verification policy should be posted on their site. This isn't as convenient as it could be, as you may have to mail in your prescription, have your doctor call, or fax the web pharmacy.

- **Where does the company do business?** Buy only from sites in the U.S. It's illegal and unsafe to buy prescription medicines from foreign sites. Look for where the company does business, and confirm that place exists. Test this by calling them up and asking for a landmark—such as a store nearby. Then, call the store and see if they can recognize the address you give them. If the company is located overseas, it is illegal and potentially dangerous to order from them. The FDA doesn't prosecute individuals, but it checks random packages at border crossings. Some Canadian pharmacies do ship reliable drugs at large savings, thanks to their government's price controls. However, this may soon change with new laws forbidding

Canadian pharmacies to accept applications from businesses that ship to the U.S.

• **Does the website have a Verified Internet Pharmacy Practice Sites seal?** This is the best way to find a safe online drugstore. The Vipps seal shows that they have been certified by the National Association of Boards of Pharmacy (NABP), a national group in Illinois that represents the 50 state pharmacy boards, as well as some international boards. To be included, a pharmacy must have good patient-pharmacist communication, must provide safe storage and shipment for its drugs, and also confirms the pharmacies' state licenses. NABP inspects their facilities. At the time of this book being written, there were only 13 Internet pharmacies with the Vipps seal, including Drugstore.com Inc. (www.drugstore.com), Eckerd.com (www.eckerd.com), and Familymeds.com (www.familymeds.com). There are other online local pharmacies that are also safe, but choose not to apply for the Vipps seal because they're not interested in operating nationwide, or their patients already have established relationships. For more information about the Vipps seal go online to www.nabp.net/vipps/intro.asp.

• **Does the pharmacy ask you to provide any personally identifiable information?** Never provide any information (such as your social security number, credit card, or medical history) unless you are confident that the site will protect it. Make sure the site does not share your information with others without your permission.

Many state medical boards and pharmacy boards are cracking down on physicians and pharmacists who prescribe and dispense drugs using only an online questionnaire. The Florida state pharmacy board is considering passing a rule to discipline pharmacists who fill prescriptions that they know are written based solely on online physician-patient interactions.

Keep in mind that your local pharmacist may be able to spot problems quickly if he knows about the other drugs you take and your medical conditions. A good Web pharmacy has pharmacists on call and requires you to fill out a questionnaire so they can flag any dangerous drug interactions.

For more information about buying drugs online, see the FDA's guide at: www.fda.gov/oc/buyonline/default.htm.

Can Cutting Your Pills Save You Money?

Many prescription drugs actually cost the same (or very close) regardless of the dosage. In other words, your 20mg pill may cost the same as a 40mg of the same prescription. Ask your doctor if they can prescribe the larger dosage. However, not all medications can be split (they may have a special coating, work on a time-release, or be in capsule form). Your doctor or pharmacist will know if you can split the pill. This will add a step to taking medicines, so be aware of this and remember to use the proper dosage. If you don't think you will remember, don't take the risk. Use the following website to calculate your savings: www.excellusbcbs.com.

Some drugstores split pills for free. It's possible to quarter pills, but most drugstores won't do this for you because pills have a tendency to crumble, and they don't want to be held liable. It's possible to get more than one month's worth of prescription at a time by splitting pills, but it depends on your insurance, number of refills, and laws in your state. If you have a flat co-pay, getting more than one month for one co-pay can save you money (but most insurances don't allow it). A way to get around this is to ask your doctor to specify in the directions to "use as directed". If you do this, make sure you know what the directed use is (for example, "1/2 tablet every morning with food"). The prescription will not say this, so don't expect the pharmacist to know.

Can Importing Drugs Save You Money?

If done properly, importing drugs can give you significant savings. Drug costs are often much lower in Canada and Mexico due to trade laws and lower manufacturing costs in those countries. For years, Americans have been visiting foreign countries to buy prescription drugs that are too expensive or unavailable in the U.S.A. As of the printing of this book, Americans are permitted to import a 90-day supply of approved drugs from these countries for personal use. The Food and Drug Administration and the U.S. Customs Service have a vague policy on the importation of unapproved and experimental drugs. Check with the Food and Drug Administration and your physician before making plans to import foreign drugs.

Drugs made and sold overseas may not have had the same manufacturing and storage standards as the same drug made in the U.S. While most drugs companies are multi-national, not all of them sell the same drugs in the same countries. The standards for storage and shelf-life of the drugs may be different. It's important to buy all of your prescription and non-prescription drugs from a reputable pharmacy. Some pharmacies may re-label drugs, sell expired pills, or even sell counterfeit pills. Be on the lookout for scams and don't buy anything if it doesn't seem right.

Drugs that are known to be abused (such as steroids, amphetamines, and some sedatives) are more tightly controlled. You should always have a copy of your doctor's prescription with you to smooth the way back. The following websites can assist you in your importing process:

www.fda.gov/ora/import/purchasing_medications.htm

www.fda.gov/ora/import/pipinfo.htm

www.customs.ustreas.gov/travel/travel.htm

Does Your Physician Have a Good Relationship with a Local Pharmacy/Pharmacist?

Once a year, bring all your drugs and nutritional supplements to your pharmacist and physician so they can suggest any less expensive alternatives. Your doctor's review should focus first on whether you still need all your medications. It's not unusual for a person to start taking a drug such as a tranquilizer for a specific symptom and to keep taking it even when it's no longer necessary.

If your doctor has a good relationship with a local pharmacist, he may be able to convince them not to charge you their highest rate (their profit margin). If you have a strong relationship with your physician or pharmacist, they will try even harder to make a situation work for you. They may have other suggestions not included in this chapter.

Often your insurance or a local law may limit your pharmacist or physician's ability to help you. A chart to help organize your findings when comparing prices can be located at www.ec-online.net/knowledge/articles/drugchart.pdf.

Good doctors will never try to push a medication on you, but even the best may not always remember your individual financial circumstances. Be sure to remind your doctor, especially when it comes to your medications, that you are trying to save money and he will almost always try to help. Most doctors have no ideas of the costs of the medications they prescribe and always try to prescribe the medication that works the best. Unfortunately, best is very subjective, as the pharmaceutical representatives who frequent the doctor's offices usually promote the newest, most expensive medications. Always ask questions about the medications you are prescribed to find out if there is a less expensive alternative.

Everyday Savings

There are many things your can do to save money on your medical bills. The number one solution is stay healthy; however, that is very unrealistic since everyone gets sick every once in a while. Just in case you don't have "healthy" genes and the best environment, here are a few pointers to help avoid those larger healthcare bills:

- Save the emergency room for emergencies.
- Avoid the hospital unless it is absolutely necessary: Over half of all health care costs are for hospital stays, and charges can be much more costly than a doctor's visit. These emergency visits also drive up your premium. Consider outpatient services and same-day surgery centers.
- Request an itemized bill (you are legally entitled to an itemized bill if you request one).
- Check out community health centers. This is a great option for the person who does not have health insurance. These clinics offer a myriad of services based on your income. You can dial 211 on your phone to find out the closest health center to you.
- If you do not have health insurance and have to go to the hospital, ask to apply for free care funds. Many hospitals throughout the country have access to private donations specifically for people who can't pay their bills. Most hospitals get reimbursed by their state for the costs of caring for people who can't pay their bills.
- Look into other local healthcare resources for check-ups and services, such as:
  - Local health departments, visiting nurses or other organizations may offer free or low-cost immunizations and screens, such as blood pressure or cholesterol checks.
  - A local dental, medical, or other health provider school may offer free or low-cost services, such as dental cleanings.
  - Your child's school may have a school-based health center or get regular visits from a medical or dental van.
  - College students may be able to get free or reduced-cost care

through their schools.

- Your local health department may know of some new programs implemented by the government recently. (You can find its number in the blue pages of your phone book.)

- Before you go in for something minor, call and speak to a doctor or nurse on the phone. Talk over your symptoms and see if you really need a visit.

- Ask if follow-up appointments are *really* necessary. Can you call and check in?

- If your doctor prescribes a medication, ask if there is a less expensive, but equally effective alternative such as a generic brand.

- Avoid unnecessary tests. Be sure you understand what tests your doctor recommends and why. Ask if every test is absolutely necessary.

- Don't pay double when you have to see another doctor or dentist. Arrange to have your records and all test results copied to your new doctor before your visit.

- Ask your doctor if s/he can give you samples of the drug you need.

- Take only the drugs you need; when your doctor prescribes a drug, be sure you understand exactly what it is for, what it is meant to do, and how long you should take it. Ask if each is absolutely necessary and how much each costs. If you are trying out a new drug, ask your doctor to prescribe only a small amount. *Do not* save prescription medications to use later, unless your doctor tells you to. Using old, leftover drugs can be dangerous.

- Look into ordering your prescriptions by mail.

- Order a 90-day supply of a prescription drug instead of a 30-day supply.

- Order drugs online, but make sure they are authentic and not substitute medications.

- Buy over-the-counter drugs when needed. Many drugs previously only available by prescription can now be found at better prices without a prescription. Ask your doctor if this will work for you.

- Look into drug company discount programs.

- Shop around for the cheaper pharmacy.

- Ask your doctor for drug discount coupons or rebates.

- Keep *all* your medical receipts—you might be eligible for a tax break. Check with the IRS, but if your medical expenses add up to more than 7.5 percent of your adjusted gross income, you may be eligible for an additional return on your taxes. Medical expenses include more than just doctor's visits and prescriptions; it may also include eyeglasses, contact lenses, physical therapy, x-rays, hearing aids, psychiatric care, insurance premiums and copays. There are phase-outs based on income, so check with the IRS at www.irs.gov.
- Obtain *all* your medical records and receipts—they may be important in applying for public programs such as Medicaid, if your bills are very high.
- Review your medical bills with a friend who is a doctor or nurse to catch unusual charges. Challenge those charges if inappropriate. It is time well spent.
- Keep yourself healthy. This is important for everyone, but never more so than when you are uninsured. Some ways to protect your health are as follows:
  - Quit smoking.
  - Use your seat belt.
  - Do not abuse alcohol or other substances. Even two drinks a day may be excessive for some people.
  - Exercise regularly; even walking does wonders.
  - Eat a low-cholesterol diet
  - Maintain a healthy weight.
  - Avoid sunburn.
  - Get enough sleep: eight hours a day.
  - Brush and floss your teeth daily.
  - Learn first aid and CPR.
  - Keep your home safe.

CHAPTER 16

NEGOTIATING WITH HEALTHCARE INSTITUTIONS AND PROVIDERS

MANY PEOPLE DON'T REALIZE that you can sometimes negotiate for lower medical bills. While this may not always work, it will never hurt to ask your doctor, hospital, or pharmacy if they're willing to come down in price.

According to the Foundation for Taxpayer and Consumer Rights (FTCR), everything in healthcare is negotiable, even the bills from your doctor, pharmacist, and hospital. FTCR's patient guide states, "You're paying the bills, not only as a consumer, but also as a taxpayer who helps fund the medical system." So don't be shy, establish the price you believe is reasonable and start negotiating!

However, before you begin your negotiations, do some research to find out what the "established price" should be. Call your insurer and ask a customer service representative how much the company will cover for the type of service you need. Then pass that information along to your doctor. If your doctor isn't willing to match the price your insurance company is willing to pay, you may want to find a physician who will. Certain insurers will even help you shop around for a doctor who will accept the insurers assignment, even if the physician is not a participating provider with your plan. This isn't as easy as it sounds because doctors and hospitals in different areas of the country charge widely varying amounts. The CMS (Centers for Medicare and Medicaid Services) website has a tool that lists how much Medicare reimburses doctors for certain medical procedures. However, the website can be rather cumbersome and hard to follow. If you go directly to www.cms.hhs.gov/apps/pfslookup/step1.asp, you will be taken to the beginning of a Medicare Physician Fee Schedule. From there, you will have to answer a series of questions in addition to knowing the HCPCS (Health Care Common Procedure Coding System) code of the procedure you are inquiring about. After you have answered these questions, a list of records will be brought up. What you will be interested in looking at are the "facility price," which means the price the doctor is reimbursed by Medicare if the procedure is performed in a hospital, and the "nonfacility price," which is the price the doctor is reimbursed by Medicare if the procedure is performed in a private doctor's office. Keep in mind that on top of these fees are other fees such as the actual "facility," equipment, pharmaceuticals, etc. which are explained in Chapter 14. Remember that this would be an estimate of a "bargain-basement prices" reserved for 39 million senior citizens and the disabled who need government assistance with their health insurance. Still, you should never pay your provider more than private insurers pay.

For example, when I was in graduate school at Georgetown University one semester, I needed to find ways to save money. Unfortunately, like most Americans, my health insurance was the first to go. However, I knew how important my annual ob-gyn visit was, especially the dreaded annual Pap smear. Since I could not afford the full physical, I decided to research what I thought would be the most expensive procedure as well as most important on my physical. To me, it was my Pap smear. Since I did not know the HCPCS code, I searched for "HCPCS Pap smear" on the Internet. Lo and behold, a myriad of articles on Pap smears appeared and, after browsing through a few of them, I found that the most recent HCPCS code was G0101 (cervical or vaginal cancer screenings; pelvic and clinical breast examination). I copied that code and then went to www.cms.hhs.gov/apps/pfslookup/step1.asp, where I answered the following questions:

1. Select the year (Example: 2006)
2. Select Healthcare Common Procedure Code (HCPC) Criteria (Example: Single HCPC Code)
3. Type of Information (Example: Pricing Information)

4.   Select Carrier option (Example: Specific Carrier)
5.   Select field options (Example: Default Fields (Pricing Information Only)
6.   HCPC (Example: G0101)
7.   Modifier (Example: All modifiers)
8.   Carrier: 00903 (Example: District of Columbia)

My pricing results came out to $41.25 "Nonfacility" and $25.42 "Facility." Since I was getting a Pap smear at my doctor's office, I targeted the Medicare rate of $41.25 when negotiating with my ob–gyn for the actual Pap smear and billed me for that rate with no hesitation, as well as giving me some sample birth control pills that I needed to carry me over until I was able to attain health insurance once again!

The reason I was able to negotiate this low price with my ob–gyn is that she knew I was a starving graduate student with no health insurance. I had been going to her for years and had always been polite, thanking her every time, sending a holiday card every year, and never asking for too much. Once I got into graduate school, she knew my income level had dropped significantly, and when I asked her about a discount, offering her $41.25 for the Pap smear instead of the regular $55. She did not hesitate to give me a break and was glad to help me out.

This is why in previous chapters I emphasized establishing a good relationship with your provider. This may seem like a trivial amount, but it can add up, especially for more expensive, surgical procedures. The better your relationship is with your provider, the more apt he or she will be willing to cut the price of you healthcare bill (i.e., it's hard to turn down a friend who asks for help who is standing right in front of you). A telephone call won't do the trick, and neither will a written request. Arrange to get "face time" with your doctor, pharmacist, or hospital billing officer and plead your own case for paying a lower amount. It also helps if you have an established relationship with your doctor or pharmacist.

Keep in mind that your provider is human too; he also has to support himself and his family and was at one point a "struggling student." So be upfront with your doctor from the initial visit. Explain to him your financial situation; mention that you pay your insurance yourself, or do not have insurance at all. He might be more compassionate than you think and try to reduce his fees for you. Just because you told his staff does not mean the doctor knows. Most doctors will work with you to help make your bill as manageable as possible.

You may also be surprised to find out that your doctor doesn't even know the precise costs of the tests and medicines he prescribes. If you find out your doctor's methods of testing are on the pricey end of the spectrum, bring this to his attention. He may do his own research and be able to suggest less expensive alternatives for the same care. Most doctors are the happiest when they make money and save you money

Another way to save money is offer to pay your doctor in cash, up front if he is willing the lower your bill to an amount that you both deem reasonable. By paying cash, the doctor is guaranteed to get your payment, and does not have to deal with the hassle of waiting for your insurance company to reimburse him, which may take months. If you don't have the cash, offer to put it on your credit card—if you're financially able to do that. Most doctor's offices will accept a markedly reduced total balance in cash (sometimes up to 50 percent discount), compared with insurance reimbursement, which often yields an even lower amount for the physician.

So, if you need care and have cash, make an offer! You will be surprised how flexible the physician may be. Exceptions to this rule usually include cosmetic plastic surgeons and dermatologists, who often do not accept insurance in the first place.

If you cannot pay cash up front, some offices may offer a payment plan, but be sure you agree to all the terms of the plan and understand them. There should be no hidden costs, such as high interest rates, that make it less expensive to use a credit card instead. for example, if you need a procedure done that costs $4,000, don't let your doctor tell you, "That's fine, but you'll have to pay the finance company $200 a month for forty months." What this means is that your doctor will get paid $3,500 by the finance company and you will eventually pay $8,000 in installments for a procedure that should have cost you only $3,500.

If you think you are going to miss a payment, call first and be honest about when you can pay under your circumstances. Most doctors are understanding and would rather help you than send you to collections. It is generally a waste of time to send your bill to collections, because it will cost at least 30 to 50 percent in legal fees (even more money than your discount) and will ruin your relationship with them. You might be surprised how much your doctor values keeping you as a patient as long as you are

dependable and honest with them. Believe it or not, many physicians actually enjoy helping people and don't practice medicine just for the money.
Hospitals, on the other hand, are a completely different story.

As described in Chapter 14, some hospitals and doctors are very creative
when it comes to their bills, and this could prove to be very exhausting on
your pocketbook. Some illegal actions taken by doctors include taking cash
payments under the table, or demanding large amounts right in the middle
of the operation and claiming that the surgery has (suddenly) turned out to
be much more complicated than they expected. Some hospitals often add a
surcharge to your bill, which may be impossible for the untrained patient to
discern.

As an individual, there is little you can do to fight this excessive goug-
ing. Fortunately, this is not what you will find 99 percent of the time. The
few doctors who do gouge their patients end up tarnishing the entire
profession. To help you avoid these pitfalls, you should refuse to deal with
pressure tactics. Demand an accurate estimate of the total (all-inclusive)
medical expenses before beginning any care, especially when planning
procedures. You should get the specific breakdown for each procedure, in
writing. for example, in the case of surgery, find out exactly what the
quoted figure covers. It should include the surgeon's fees, the assistant's
charges, anesthesia, operation theatre charges, hospitalization expenses, post-
operative care, and follow-up visits.

If you are having a procedure done at a hospital, your doctor may be able
to help you work something out with the hospital administration. Unfortunately, when people seek treatment from a hospital, they are billed with "list
prices" that the hospital claims that they can't negotiate. But this isn't true.
The Department of Health and Human Services has directed all 4,800 hospitals in the United States to negotiate with patients on services. And most
doctors are aware of this. If the doctor is unable to work out a deal with the
hospital, ask the doctor whom you should talk to at the hospital in order to
negotiate a lower cost. Let that person know that you want to work out a
payment plan based on the "Medicare rate." That is the target you should
are shooting for. Hospitals are bureaucratic organizations and they will try
to bill you as much as they can. But you can work this in your favor. If the
hospital is unwilling to negotiate their charges, your doctor may be able to
lessen his own charges, and you might save up to 40 percent. A good rule of
thumb is to try never to pay more than what an HMO (or your local

government) has negotiated as the set price for a specific service. This is especially the case if you are going to the doctor's private clinic.

If you are having a procedure done at a hospital, be sure to do the following at least one week before the surgery to decrease your final bill:

- If you know you are going to have surgery, call each of the hospitals you are considering and ask their policies on discounts for payment in advance. Some hospitals give a percentage discount and some a flat fee. Flat fees are usually a better deal, and usually include the anesthesiology charge as well. Select a surgeon who has privileges at the hospital, or find out if your surgeon is willing to seek courtesy privileges at that hospital.

- Your doctor will identify the exact surgery he plans to do and place it on the operating schedule, approximately one week before the scheduled date. When you talk to you doctor or the surgeon's nurse who does the scheduling, ask to be scheduled first or second case on the date he proposes; this gives you more time to fool with the billing folks before they get busy, and gets you out of the hospital quicker.

- Call the hospital accounting office as soon as you know the case has been scheduled. Tell them you want to discuss prepayment for a self-pay surgery. Tell them you are scheduled for "name exact surgery" with "name doctor" on "date". Get the full name of the bookkeeping person you talk to. Ask if there is a set fee or discount if you pay in full, in advance on the day of the surgery. Write down the exact amount and the name of the person you talked to and ask them to make sure it is put on your record that you are eligible for the advance payment rate.

- Ask what is included. For example, I wanted to go have my EKG and labs the day before (so I wouldn't have to get up so early), but the bookkeeper told me that these tests were included in the fee if I had them done the morning of surgery, but would be billed separately if I did them another day. For $400, I got up early!

- Ask what the discount for the additional room fee is (if you have to stay overnight). Some hospitals do not discount this part. Most do.

- Ask where the information about your prepayment arrangement is being recorded for the admitting clerk.

- Make sure that the fees quoted include the anesthesiology and pathology fees. Insist on including these as they can often end up costing as much as the procedure itself!
- Ask if the hospital accepts Visa or MasterCard and if the same rate applies. The answer is usually yes, and you can really rack up the frequent-flyer miles.

The day of your surgery, take the written bookkeeping clerk's name and agreed amount with you:

- Take a credit card or two checks with you.
- Arrive at least 15 minutes ahead of when they said; sign in right away.
- Write down the admitting clerk's name, and call her or him by name. Tell the clerk as soon as she asks about insurance that you are self-pay and that you have made a payment agreement for (flat rate) or (discounted) prepayment with "name," who told you the information would be recorded.
- Give them the check or credit card and get a receipt.
- If something unusual or unexpected happens, make sure the agreement gets written into your records. I planned to pay by Master-Card, and their machine was broken. They told me to come back after surgery before I left the hospital, when they could use another department's machine. I told them I was there early, ready to pay, and that I would be too ill to come back after the surgery, I would need to go home. They said to send a family member later. I reminded them that no one else could sign the charge slip. I asked them why they couldn't bring it to me in postrecovery, and they said they could. I told them to make sure that it was written in my record that I was ready to pay and entitled to the discounted prepay agreement. Sure enough, they did not follow through, and I left without signing the receipt. I went back a few days later after my surgeon's visit, and if I had not had the agreement written on the record, they would have charged me the full amount.
- Because not many people use the prepayment option, the bookkeeping isn't very successful, and the chances are good—fifty-fifty—that you will still get a full bill showing a balance due. Do not

ignore it! Call the person you originally talked to, who gave you the rate, and remind him or her of your conversation, say you were incorrectly billed, and ask the person to fix it and send you a corrected copy. Hospitals are very quick to send patients to collections, often after the third unanswered bill.

- You may still receive a few smaller separate bills for pathologist and radiologist professional fees. It's hard to get a prepaid discount on these, but some do discount 10 or 20 percent for payment in full within 30 days. As soon as you get these bills, call the office! Ask!

On the other hand, if you have a procedure done and have lost track of your bills, you can end up with a large bill at your door right before it's sent to collections. In this case, call your doctor immediately and offer to pay half the bill in cash immediately. Nine out of ten times your offer will be accepted (if the bill goes to collections, the doctor will receive only 50 percent anyway because the law firm's commission is 50 percent).

Another easy way to shave money from your bill is to always ask your doctor if there is a less expensive, but equally effective, alternative drug. Sometimes an over-the-counter product will fit what you are looking for. There are many drugs that were formerly available only with a prescription that can now be found at lower prices without a prescription—but at lower dosages.

It pays to ask your doctor to help. Your doctor might also have connections with a pharmaceutical company. He may be able to provide you with some samples to get you started, or even be able to call and get you an extra discount. Some doctors even have good relationships with the pharmacies they call into frequently. A pharmacy that is anxious to get more business could offer your doctor extra discounts that leave more cash in your pockets.

If you have to get a procedure done that requires an overnight stay at a hospital, be sure to ask the doctor which hospital that he prefers and which is least expensive. As before, some doctors may not know specific costs, but if they practice at 3 different hospitals in the are and say that all are equally as good, do a little more research and find out how much each hospital charges per day per bed (in other words, per a night at the hospital). Some emergency rooms differ drastically in cost, so price checking before an emergency happens may save you money in the future. And often, ambulatory surgical centers are *much less* expensive than most hospitals, and should be preferred for otherwise healthy patients.

If you have a good relationship with your doctor, you may also be able to save money on your visits. Instead of going in every time you need a refill on a prescription or get sick, you may be able to call the office and tell the doctor's receptionist or nurse your symptoms and your pharmacy number. They can let your doctor know. If it's necessary for you to come in, you will get a call back; otherwise, your doctor can call in the prescription you need without the hassle—or charge—of a visit. Whenever you do this, it's a good idea to say thank you the next time you see your doctor so they don't think you are taking advantage of them.

Your doctor can save you a great deal of financial headaches if you befriend him. Most doctors go into the medical field because they enjoy helping people. If you ask, you may be pleasantly surprised by how your doctor can help you. He or she can be your biggest ally in your time of need.

CONCLUSION

WHY IS HEALTHCARE SO EXPENSIVE? This is the million dollar question. Some of its costs we are able to reduce, but others are out of our hands entirely. Newer and costlier medical technologies, pharmaceuticals, and treatments clearly play a key role in driving up costs, but so do frivolous malpractice suits, bad choices, and just the lack of knowing the details of your own health.

While we have no control over some parts of this, we do have control over our own medical bills. As consumers, we have the information and resources we need to make more economical choices. We have the ability to choose treatments that fit our situation. Don't allow the healthcare system to dictate what your treatment will be! You are an individual who has choices. Do you let the car sales person tell you which car you can buy, or do you do the research and select the best one for you?

Once you have read this book, you are on your way to saving money on your healthcare. Ask yourself the following questions to see if you are actually saving as much as possible:

1. Do you trust your doctor?
2. Have you ever negotiated with your doctor?
3. Do you know all the options in your health plan—and those in newer plans?
4. Do you practice preventative care and know how does your insurance define preventative care?
5. Do you know what a medical bill looks like and do you understand it?
6. Do you know what you can do today that will save you money on your medical bills tomorrow?

For every question you were unable to answer affirmatively, you have lost hundreds and possibly even thousands of dollars on your healthcare.

Trust Your Doctor

Your relationship with your doctor is one of the most important parts of maintaining your health. We're talking about a very personal relationship—one that requires your comfort while discussing sensitive issues and a relationship that could last a lifetime. Your job is to identify the factors that are most important to YOU—gender, ethnicity, age, marital status, whether they have children, and sexual orientation can all play a part in your comfort and ability to talk openly with your doctor. In Part I, we identified how to find this person as well as how to communicate with them most effectively.

Your relationship with your primary care physician is one of the most important things to consider in your healthcare. I am personally a big believer in continuity, and because of that, believe that a doctor who has seen you repeatedly over the years has a much better understanding of how your immediate health issues relates to your past health issues. If you hit a bump in the road with your current physician, I would suggest trying to work on your relationship instead of immediately changing doctors. Times like these may even allow you to strengthen your relationship with a trusted caregiver.

Negotiate with Your Doctor

You may have negotiated a decent price on your new car, house, or even bargained for a night stand from your neighbor's yard sale. It shouldn't come as a surprise to you that you can negotiate down your healthcare as well. After reading the chapter "Negotiating with Your Doctor," you should have the information you need to effectively haggle with your doctor to lower your out-of-pocket expenses. Start comparing prices, come up with a price that is reasonable, and ask for it. Would you buy a car at the first price the salesperson gave you? Go ahead and give a counteroffer. Use the guidelines below to accomplish this effectively. Remember: The choice is yours.

- Find out what others are paying.
- Ask for the best price.
- Cash talks (so do credit cards).
- Payment plans option.
- Don't avoid the bill.
- Plead your own case.
- If you don't have health insurance, let your doctor know.
- If you have an on-going or recurring medical problem, ask your doctor if he/she can phone-in a prescription without a visit.

If you keep all of these points in mind, you should have no problem negotiating your medical bill. Unfortunately, if you are a Medicare recipient, or on co-payments and deductibles, it's rare that you will be able to successfully negotiate a lower rate, but it is possible. Kudos to you if you accomplish this.

Knowing Your Health Insurance Options

The same doctor you trust to give you the best healthcare suggestions may also be able to steer you in the right direction when it comes to health insurance. In Part II, we discussed your health insurance and gave you the tools you need to help you make wise choices in healthcare.

Today's healthcare costs are high, and premiums seem to be increasing without covering as much. You buy health insurance for the same reason you buy other kinds of insurance: to protect yourself financially. With health insurance, you need to read the fine print and be sure you will be getting what you need. You can't always predict what your medical bills will be from year to year, and you need to prioritize what you want and need from your health plan to determine what type is best for you and your family. Below are a few things to consider:

- Are you a "young family"?
- Do you have college age kids?
- Are you healthy adults?
- Do you travel for work?
- Do you or anyone in your family have ongoing medical concerns?
- Do you need urgent or emergency coverage?
- How well do you budget your money?
- Do you want to have the freedom of choosing your own doctors?
- Do you mind paperwork?
- Do you prefer a plan that includes routine and preventive care?
- Do you need group or individual insurance?
- How much will the plan cost you?
- What type and level of service do you expect for the price you will be paying?
- What are the extra "bells and whistles"?
- What do other subscribers say about the plan or the company?

Selecting a healthcare plan can feel overwhelming, so be sure to take your time. Depending on what plan you are interested in, your rights are different, based on how you get your coverage, the type of plan you have (HMO, PPO, Point of Service,etc.), and your state of residence. You can get information about agencies in your state that can help you resolve a problem you may be having by visiting www.healthinsuranceinfo.net or by obtaining general consumer information on health insurance at www.healthcarecoach.com. Take your time when deciding on an insurance plan. There is no sense getting a healthcare policy that will not cover you when you really need it for those big hospital bills.

Preventative Care

Even when you have a health plan, you shouldn't be reckless with your body. For example, if you have a family history of breast cancer, you may want to consult you doctor on considering your first mammograms earlier than the normal age of 40. By initiating this exam earlier, you will become more aware of what is considered normal and what is not, and will be able to report something unusual before it potentially becomes more serious. This will save you far more money and potentially save your life if it was caught early enough. Some local healthcare clinics have programs that will provide uninsured women with free breast and cervical cancer screens (even treatment, if necessary). Check around your local area to find ways to monitor your health and prevent illnesses, instead of merely reacting to them.

In general, you should try to stay as healthy as possible, so your body does not start falling apart at a fragile point. Make sure to work out a schedule of preventive health screenings with your doctor that is appropriate for your age and gender. The lower your medical bills are, the lower your premiums will be. Some healthcare companies have Adolescent Immunization Reminders sent to parents of 12-year-olds encouraging regular checkups, management for certain diseases, discounts to community-based weight loss programs, home exercise equipment, etc. Be sure to make good lifestyle choices such as avoid smoking a pack of cigarettes a day.

Understand Your Medical Bill

When you receive bills from the hospital or doctor, always check to make sure they accurately reflect what you have undergone and take your insurance into consideration. Some errors, such as wrong computer codes, are common, and you may be billed for healthcare you never received. These days, most hospitals have "patient advocacy" groups that will help with these issues and are sure that they are properly resolved before it is too late. Often times, if an unanticipated complication occurs in the course of your care, the hospital will gladly give a discount rather than face a potential malpractice claim.

Pay special attention to the most common areas of overcharges and errors, plus any irregularities in your medical records and itemized bill, for example:

- Duplicate billing
- Duplication of tests
- Number of days in hospital
- Incorrect room charges
- Operating room time
- Upcoding
- Keystroke error
- Canceled work
- Services never rendered
- Erroneous charges

It feels like hospitals discourage you from examining your bills too closely. Please be proactive and don't leave this up to your insurance companies. If your hospitalization wasn't for an emergency, check your insurance policy ahead of time to find out just what it will cover and how much it will pay. Be sure to carefully review the section on "exceptions and exclusions." It will tell you what your plan will not cover.

Everyday Savings

Pay attention to what you may do or don't do for your health on a daily basis. For example, before you go to your local pharmacy to pick up a prescription ask yourself these questions:

- Do I really need this?
- Can I get something as comparable as this over-the-counter?
- Is there a generic form of this prescription?
- Did my doctor write me a prescription for the maximum amount that I can get with my co-pay?

- Is this pharmacy charging me the same amount as the one across the street? Is there a BJs, Costco, or Priceclub nearby where I can get my prescription cheaper?
- Am I eligible for a drug discount program or any government drug program?

Don't forget the everyday health questions such as:
- Do I really need this cigarette?
- When is the last time I went in for a check-up?
- When is the last time I did something active, like jog?
- Do I know my doctor's first name? Do I know what my doctor looks like?
- What is my doctor's nurse's name? My technician's? My receptionist's?
- Do I know how to contact my doctor in case of an emergency, or to ask if I need to go to the emergency room?
- Where is the closest clinic?
- When is the last time I called my state department of health to find out what new healthcare programs were available to people like me try to save money on my healthcare?
- Have I reviewed my healthcare benefits in the last year?
- Does my insurance plan still exist?
- Has my legal status changed within this past year due to marriage, kids, divorce, or taking care of a relative?
- Did I write off any healthcare benefits on my taxes?

The above are just a handful of questions you can ask yourself every day to maintain your savings on a day-to-day basis. If you need more information, reread Chapter 15. You might be able to save yourself a headache and a few dollars—or maybe more.

At the end of the day, what have we learned? Spend more time choosing your doctor, choose a health plan that works for you, stay healthy and practice preventative care, ask the right questions, and review your medical bills carefully. These simple steps are all you need to take to save you thousands of dollars every year.

Appendix A:
Medical Test Checklist

You should fill out this checklist for every medical test suggested and keep track of all the "preventive" tests you may have had earlier. Chapter 13 went over some of the preventive tests and what could be applied to a basic screening of a potential diagnosis, instead of having to retake a preventive test that might be costly.

Test name _____

_____

Description _____

_____

Purpose _____

_____

To confirm diagnosis? _____ Diagnosis _____

To exclude diagnosis? _____ Diagnosis _____

Where will the test be done? Clinic? _____

Independent lab? _____ Hospital? _____

Cost of test in: Clinic _____ Independent lab _____

Hospital _____

Are there risks associated with the test (i.e., is the test invasive)? ____
_____

If yes, what risks? _____
_____

Are there less invasive tests that might give the same information?
_____
_____

If the test result is abnormal, what will be done next? _____
_____

If the rest result is normal, what will be done? _____
_____

Comments _____
_____
_____
_____
_____
_____
_____
_____
_____
_____
_____

Sample Worksheet for Making Medical Decisions About Treatments				
	Option 1	Option 2	Option 3	Option 4
Benefits:				
Success:				
Risks:				
Costs:				
Time:				
Decision (in the rank of choice):				
What to do if medical insurance rejects preferred treatment:				

Appendix B:
Questions to Ask
a Potential Doctor

Below is a brief checklist you might want to ask the office manager or other staff in addition to other questions you may have. Some of these items may be better answered by your health plan than with the doctor's office.

Which hospitals does the doctor use?

Doctor A: _____

_____

Doctor B: _____

_____

Doctor C: _____

_____

What are the office hours (when is the doctor available and when can I speak to office staff)?

Doctor A: _____

_____

Doctor B: _____

_____

Doctor C: _____

_____

Does the doctor or someone else in the office speak the language that I am most comfortable speaking?

Doctor A: _____

_____

Doctor B: _____

_____

Doctor C: _____

_____

How many other doctors "cover" for the doctor when he or she is not available? Who are they?

Doctor A: _____

_____

Doctor B: _____

_____

Doctor C: _____

_____

How long does it usually take to get a routine appointment?

Doctor A: _____

_____

Doctor B: _____

_____

Doctor C: _____

_____

How long might I need to wait in the office before seeing the doctor?

Doctor A: _____

_____

Doctor B: _____

_____

Doctor C: _____

_____

What happens if I need to cancel an appointment? Will I have to pay for it anyway?

Doctor A: _____

_____

Doctor B: _____

_____

Doctor C: _____

_____

Does the office send reminders about prevention tests, for example, Pap smears?

Doctor A: _____

_____

Doctor B: _____

_____

Doctor C: _____

_____

What do I do if I need urgent care or have an emergency?

Doctor A: _____

_____

Doctor B: _____

_____

Doctor C: _____

_____

Does the doctor (or a nurse or physician assistant) give advice over the phone for common medical problems?

Doctor A: _____

_____

Doctor B: _____

_____

Doctor C: _____

_____

You may also want to talk briefly with the doctor by phone or in person. Ask if you are able to do this and if there is a charge.

Appendix C: Glossary

Benefits: The medical services included in a health insurance policy to which the insured person or persons are entitled.

Calendar year: The time period from January 1 to December 31 in a single year.

Catastrophic health insurance: Insurance, with a very high deductible, covering an injury or illness with medical expenses that are above the normal parameters of basic health insurance.

Claim: A health-related bill submitted for payment to a health insurance company by the policy holder or healthcare provider.

COBRA: "Consolidated Omnibus Budget Reconciliation Act" of 1985 is a regulation that affects most U.S. employers of over 20 employees, whereby they must offer departing employees a continuation of their health insurance; it includes other options.

Coinsurance: The percentage of costs (usually 20 percent) that a patient pays after the deductible is met. Coinsurance is most commonly found in the indemnity, fee-for-service and PPO markets, but not in the HMO market.

Copayment or copay: A cost sharing arrangement in which the insured or enrollee pays a specific flat dollar amount to the provider, usually for each specific service. The most common percentage copayment is 20 percent. A common copay is $5 to $15 per visit.

Coverage: A health care service that qualifies as a benefit under the terms of an insurance contract.

Deductible: The set dollar amount that a subscriber must pay before insurance coverage for medical expenses can begin. A typical deductible amount may be several hundred dollars to several thousand per year, depending on the insurance policy.

Discount plans: Large buying organizations formed to provide discounts on health services to its members. It is not a form of health insurance.

Drug benefits: It is extremely important to find out all the terms of the plan before enrolling. For example, some plans limit or don't even include drug benefits. Some have high deductibles and some provide limited reimbursement. Drug benefits can be costly if not covered by the plan.

Family health insurance: Health coverage taking into account the unique needs in each family. It can be either a group or an individual type of insurance.

Group health insurance: Health coverage based on a group of people, whether assembled by an organization or a business. The cost is spread out among the members of the group. Under federal guidelines, a "large employer" is one with 51 or more employees and a "small employer" averages 2 to 50 employees in a calendar year.

HIPAA: Health Insurance Portability and Accountability Act; gives patients a means to consult the documents that pertain to their medical care; provides that a person with a preexisting condition, who has had continuous health coverage for more than 12 months, can leave a job and not be turned down for health insurance at a new job.

HMO: Health maintenance organization, a type of group health plan in which an organization is formed to provide medical care to its members. The physicians and medical personnel work for the HMO and provide medical care to the members of the HMO, with limited referrals to outside specialists. There is often an emphasis on prevention of disease and participation in programs for better health. Recently, members of HMOs may see healthcare professionals outside of their system, with higher fees. Members usually obtain all of their medical needs from their HMO clinics through managed medical care.

HSA: Health savings account, a personal savings account set up to be used exclusively for medical expenses and is paired with a high deductible health insurance policy.

Individual health insurance: Health coverage on an individual basis, not part of a group. The premium is usually higher for individual health insurance than for a group policy.

Managed care: Comprehensive healthcare which is provided to participating members of an organized healthcare organization through the use of a network of healthcare providers and facilities; it uses a delivery system that secures cost effective healthcare.

Maximum limits: The highest dollar amounts a health insurance plan will pay: 1) for a single claim; 2) over the lifetime of an insured person.

Network: The doctors or other medical providers and facilities that either work for or contract with a group healthcare organization.

Out-of-network: Doctors or other medical providers and facilities which either do not work for or which do not contract with a group healthcare organization.

Out-of-pocket maximum or maximum payout: The limit of the amount you have to pay each year for covered services when you have reached the maximum amount. If you receive health benefits from your employer, your benefits manager, or your human resources department should be able to help you understand your benefits and the definitions as well as your responsibilities. If your employer can't help, ask if there is an insurance agent you can call

PCP: Primary care physician or personal care provider, a physician or other medical care provider who participates in a healthcare system. As previously emphasized, it is important to build a good working relationship with your primary care physician. The health plan may call this person your primary care physician (PCP), gatekeeper, or family doctor. This person will take care of most of your medical needs and will the person to refer you to a specialist if deemed necessary by your insurance provider and/or PCP, as well as specify who has the final say and who has the authority to deny or approve your doctor's request. Terms of referrals should be referenced in the EOC or SPD. If they are not, be sure they are outlined for you before you select a provider.

Policy: The legal agreement between an insurance company and insured person, whereby the company agrees to pay for the covered medical services included in the agreement and the insured agrees to pay the premium price.

POS: Point of service, a type of group insurance with a combination of HMO and PPO characteristics. The policyholders must use a primary care physician, but they can use other network health providers when needed or go to out-of-network providers, at higher cost.

PPO: Preferred provider organization, a type of group health plan. The medical professionals in the system agree to accept a standard fee schedule and patient care controls; the system is usually organized by an insurance company. In a PPO, the policyholder can go to any medical provider in the PPO network and pay the copayment amount for each regular service. If the policyholder chooses to go to an out-of-network provider, he or she often pays that doctor's fees directly and files for reimbursement from the insurance company. This is a greater cost. For that reason, the PPO system encourages its policyholders to see the doctors and health care providers who are part of the system.

Preexisting condition: A physical or mental condition that existed before applying for a policy, for which medical care was already recommended or received, and which may not be covered by insurance, or only after a time lapse.

Premium: The money paid by an insured person or business for a health insurance policy.

Prescription plan: An organized plan whereby prescription needs are provided to group members at a lower cost, usually through a vendor with a pharmacy network that covers the whole country and negotiates for lower drug costs.

Provider: A physician, hospital, medical care facility, or other type of medical personnel who provides healthcare.

Referral: The method whereby a physician directs a patient to the services of another physician.

SDHP: Self-directed health plan; utilizes a money account with a declining balance used for medical expenses.

SOS (Help): You can call the customer service phone number listed in your EOC or SPD. Ask the health plan representative to explain the specific policy, benefit, limitation or further define the above definitions in relevance to their plan. If you purchased your own health insurance, call the insurance broker who sold you the policy or ask your health plan for help in understanding what is covered and not covered. If all else fails, you may want to call an agency such as the Health Insurance Counseling and Advocacy Program (HICAP), which provides information and assistance with Medicare, managed care (HMOs), long-term care insurance, and other health insurance issues and can help answer. You can find your local center online at www.inlandagency.org/html/ hicap_otherstates.htm.

Appendix D:
Your Personal Health History

Use this form to keep track of your health history. Print out a copy and take it with you to your doctor appointments to help keep you and your doctor up-to-date.

1. I was in the hospital for (list conditions):   Date

_____

_____

_____

_____

_____

2. I have had these surgeries: Date

_____

_____

_____

_____

3. I have had these injuries/conditions/illnesses: Date

_____

_____

_____

_____

4. I have these allergies (list type of allergy — food, medicine, etc. — and reaction):

_____

_____

_____

_____

_____

5. I have had these immunizations (shots):
   (Note: In the list below, the names of the shots follow the names of the diseases they prevent.)

For children:	Suggested age	Date(s) received
Hepatitis B (HBV)	Dose 1: Birth to 2 months	_____
	Dose 2: 2 months to 4 months	_____
	Dose 3: 6 months to 18 months	_____
	Dose 1 or 3: 11 years to 12 years	_____
Polio (IPV)	Dose 1: 2 months	_____
	Dose 2: 4 months	_____
	Dose 3: 6 months to 18 months	_____
	Dose 4: 4 years to 6 years	_____
Haemophilus Influenzae type B (Hib)		
	Dose 1: 2 months	_____
	Dose 2: 4 months	_____
	Dose 3: 6 months	_____
	Dose 4: 12 months to 15 months	_____
Diphtheria, Tetanus, & Pertussis (DTaP, Td)		
	Dose 1: 2 months	_____
	Dose 2: 4 months	_____
	Dose 3: 6 months	_____
	Dose 4: 15 months to 18 months	_____
	Dose 5: 4 years to 6 years	_____
	Td Once: 11 years to 16 years	_____

Measles, Mumps, Rubella (MMR)

Dose 1: 12 months to 15 months _____

Dose 2: 4 years to 6 years _____

or Dose 2: 11 years to 12 years _____

Chickenpox (Varicella) (VZV)

Once: 12 months to 18 months _____

or once: 11 years to 12 years _____

Pneumococcal Disease (Prevnar™)

Dose 1: 2 months _____

Dose 2: 4 months _____

Dose 3: 6 months _____

Dose 4: 12 months to 15 months _____

Hepatitis A

Once: 2 years to 12 years _____
in selected areas

For adults:	Suggested age	Date(s) received
Influenza	Every year starting at age 65	_____
Pneumococcal	Once at age 65	_____
Tetanus (Td)	Every 10 years	_____

6. I take these medicines/supplements (bring with you, if possible):

_____

_____

_____

_____

_____

7. My family members (parents, brothers, sisters, grandparents) have/had these major conditions:

_____

_____

_____

_____

_____

8. I see these other health care providers:

Name   Why I see them

_____   _____

_____   _____

_____   _____

_____   _____

_____   _____

Appendix E:
Hospital Checklist

Reason for Admission (Diagnosis) _____
_____
_____
_____

What procedures, tests or treatments cannot be done as an outpatient?
_____
_____
_____
_____

What tests could be done prior to admission to shorten hospital stay?
_____
_____
_____
_____

Expected length of stay (days) _____

Choice of hospitals: _____
_____
_____
_____

Hospital Average Daily Cost: _____
_____Rs_____
_____Rs_____
_____Rs_____

Can admission be arranged early in the morning (rather than the previous night, thus helping to reduce your bill)?
_____
_____

Are consultations planned? _____
_____
_____

If yes, why, and who will perform them? _____
_____
_____

Can the consultants be seen prior to admission? _____
_____
_____

If diagnosis or treatment is unclear, has specialty consultation been considered? _____
_____
_____
_____

If not, why not?_____
_____
_____
_____

COMMENTS

_____

_____

Daily Hospital Checklist

Reason for continued hospitalization? _____

_____

_____

_____

What procedures, tests, or treatments cannot be done as an outpatient? ___

_____

_____

_____

Tests ordered today: _____

_____

_____

Tests needed before discharge: _____

_____

_____

Medications:

Medications ordered today?	How often?	Why
_____	_____	_____
_____	_____	_____
_____	_____	_____
_____	_____	_____

Can any medications be stopped? (Go over list): _____

_____

_____

Can I eat (or eat more): _____

_____

_____

Can IV be removed? _____

_____

_____

Can I walk around? _____

_____

_____

What extra hospital equipment is presently in use: _____

_____

_____

_____

Can any procedures the use of any or equipment be discontinued? ___

_____

_____

_____

_____

_____

How many physicians continue to be involved with care? _____

_____

Who? _____

_____

Why? _____

_____

Discharge Plans

When? _____

Where? _____

Will additional nursing care be needed at home?_____
_____

Has this been arranged? _____
_____

Has transportation home been arranged? _____
_____

When do I see the doctor after being discharged? _____

Where? _____

Whom do I contact if I have a medical problem? _____
_____

Whom do I contact if I have a problem with the hospital bill? _____
_____
_____
_____

Appendix F:
Sample Bills

This detailed bill demonstrates how important it is to listen to your doctor when they explain what is going to happen during the procedure—and take notes. This bill is for a routine colonoscopy and endoscopy. Some samples were taken.

If the questions asked had only covered how the procedure went, the doctor may have only answered: "It went fine. The biopsies came back normal." You must, however, ask more detailed questions in order to confirm the accuracy of the bill; for example, "How many samples were taken?" is a good question.

If you do not ask these questions of your doctor, you can always ask the billing department directly to explain the bill and query what each charge is for. You should not be expected to catch the mistakes on your own, and your doctor, in most cases, will not have the time to explain. By going to the billing department, you may catch the billing department noticing a miscoded charge.

There are a few mistakes in this bill. When a doctor does an endoscopy or colonoscopy, they do not need a "path stain grp1" because it is already included in the "surg path lev IV". It is normal to be charged individually for the samples taken, but please confirm that the number of samples is correct. The second mistake lies in the charging of both "bio during colon"/"bio during endo" and the "disposable snare". It should be either/or.

Again, it is important to the billing department with your questions. It is their job to explain what was done until you understand it, and if they are having a difficult time explaining, it is probably because they do not understand it themselves. In that case, they should return to your file and query the doctor directly.

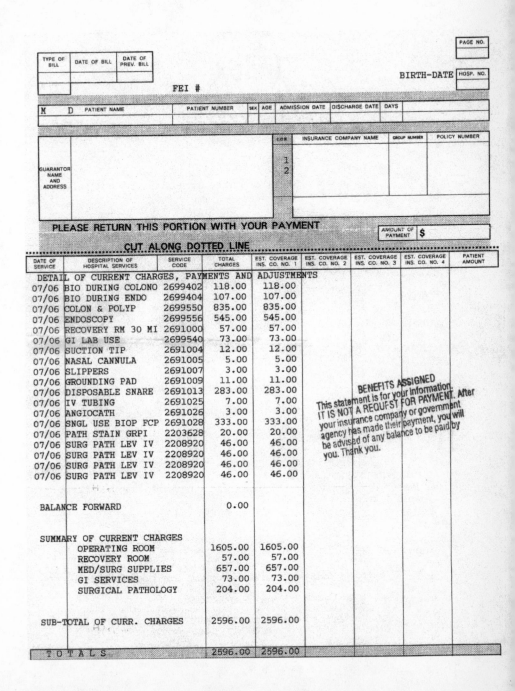

					PAGE NO.

TYPE OF BILL	DATE OF BILL	DATE OF PREV. BILL		BIRTH-DATE	HOSP. NO.
			FEI #		

M	D	PATIENT NAME	PATIENT NUMBER	SEX	AGE	ADMISSION DATE	DISCHARGE DATE	DAYS	

			C.O.B	INSURANCE COMPANY NAME	GROUP NUMBER	POLICY NUMBER
GUARANTOR NAME AND ADDRESS			1 2			

PLEASE RETURN THIS PORTION WITH YOUR PAYMENT

AMOUNT OF PAYMENT $

CUT ALONG DOTTED LINE

DATE OF SERVICE	DESCRIPTION OF HOSPITAL SERVICES	SERVICE CODE	TOTAL CHARGES	EST. COVERAGE INS. CO. NO. 1	EST. COVERAGE INS. CO. NO. 2	EST. COVERAGE INS. CO. NO. 3	EST. COVERAGE INS. CO. NO. 4	PATIENT AMOUNT
	DETAIL OF CURRENT CHARGES, PAYMENTS AND ADJUSTMENTS							
07/06	BIO DURING COLONO	2699402	118.00	118.00				
07/06	BIO DURING ENDO	2699404	107.00	107.00				
07/06	COLON & POLYP	2699550	835.00	835.00				
07/06	ENDOSCOPY	2699556	545.00	545.00				
07/06	RECOVERY RM 30 MI	2691000	57.00	57.00				
07/06	GI LAB USE	2699540	73.00	73.00				
07/06	SUCTION TIP	2691004	12.00	12.00				
07/06	NASAL CANNULA	2691005	5.00	5.00				
07/06	SLIPPERS	2691007	3.00	3.00				
07/06	GROUNDING PAD	2691009	11.00	11.00				
07/06	DISPOSABLE SNARE	2691013	283.00	283.00				
07/06	IV TUBING	2691025	7.00	7.00				
07/06	ANGIOCATH	2691026	3.00	3.00				
07/06	SNGL USE BIOP FCP	2691028	333.00	333.00				
07/06	PATH STAIN GRPI	2203628	20.00	20.00				
07/06	SURG PATH LEV IV	2208920	46.00	46.00				
07/06	SURG PATH LEV IV	2208920	46.00	46.00				
07/06	SURG PATH LEV IV	2208920	46.00	46.00				
07/06	SURG PATH LEV IV	2208920	46.00	46.00				
	BALANCE FORWARD		0.00					
	SUMMARY OF CURRENT CHARGES							
	OPERATING ROOM		1605.00	1605.00				
	RECOVERY ROOM		57.00	57.00				
	MED/SURG SUPPLIES		657.00	657.00				
	GI SERVICES		73.00	73.00				
	SURGICAL PATHOLOGY		204.00	204.00				
	SUB-TOTAL OF CURR. CHARGES		2596.00	2596.00				
	TOTALS		2596.00	2596.00				

BENEFITS ASSIGNED
This statement is for your information.
IT IS NOT A REQUEST FOR PAYMENT. After
your insurance company or government
agency has made their payment, you will
be advised of any balance to be paid by
you. Thank you.

Index

R

Railroad Retirement Board
(RRB), 87

rectal exam, 156

referral, 213

Religious Fraternal Benefit (RFB)
Society Plans, 100

research your options, 52–56

respecting your doctor and staff,
17–18

S

samples, using, 174–175

saving suggestions, 185–188

scheduling a visit, 13–15

screening tests, recommended
for men, 154–157
women, 158–160

second opinions
checklist for your visit,
33–35
decision-making, 35–37,
38–40
research your options,
40–41
role of, 30
sources of, 32–33

when to get a second
opinion, 31–32

selecting your healthcare plan
beginning your search,
45–47

broker, using a, 48–49

COBRA, 52

comparing plans, 50–52

denial of coverage, 59–60

FFS, 51

finding a plan in your area,
47–48

FSAs/HSAs/HRAs, 52

Health Insurance
Portability and
Accountability Act of
1996 (HIPPA), 57, 58

HMOs, 51

Medicaid, 51–52

Medicare, 51

POS, 51

PPOs, 51

preexisting conditions, 57,
58

research your options,
52–56

TRICARE, 52

V

W